Exercising With Purpose

Written By: Linton McClain

Cover Art By: Linton McClain

Photographer: Agnes Lopez

This book is dedicated to my mother- who taught me the true value of integrity

Contents

Acknowledgments 6

Preface 7

Introduction 10

Step One **Finding Purpose** 23

Step Two **Setting Goals** 47

Step Three **Body Types** 63

Step Four **Exercise Routine** 71

Step Five **Proper Nutrition** 109

Step Six **Journals** 125

Step Seven **Obstacles** 133

Step Eight **Exercising with Others** 155

Step Nine **Staying Focused** 163

Works Cited 174

Index 175

About the Author 177

Acknowledgments

I would like to thank my family and friends, for encouraging me to be the best and extending their ever-present support.

I would like to give a personal thanks to my mentors, Larry Shivertaker and Karin Deleuran. You have both challenged me to go above and beyond my abilities, and helped me stay the course necessary to finish this manual. You have helped me accomplish many feats, and I just want you to know that your work is just beginning.

To everyone I have had the honor of teaching my training philosophy; you have given me the spark I needed to keep my engine running. You help me strive to achieve more each and every day. You all motivate me daily and continue to inspire me.

To the children all around the world; may we be reminded through their innocence of what it means to enjoy life, and live for the moment. May we all be humbled and appreciate the real treasures of life.

Preface

Have you ever been in a position in which you wanted to achieve a specific exercise goal; but there was no one available to give you the education or guidance? You attempt to achieve your goals alone, only to frustrate yourself because it is boring, time consuming, and it does not seem work for you. Maybe you want to stay in shape but realize you are just burned out from practicing the same routine over and over again? Maybe you are the type of person who has exercised for so long that you do not know how to enjoy it anymore. After training and coaching individuals to stay healthy and fit for over 9 years, I have discovered one thing common among those who struggle daily with the never ending battle of staying in shape: lack of proper motivation and guidance.

At this day and age, we are well aware of the benefits of exercising. In fact, we are reminded daily of the repercussions of being sedentary: obesity, loss of mobility, and chronic health conditions. With all of the knowledge and visual stimulation, why is it that most individuals would choose not to have a healthy and functioning body? You do not have to think about this one. I will say it for you. We have priorities in our life that supersede our health. For example, we understand the importance of eating, taking the car to the shop, or showing up to work on time. We make time for these events without question. Is it not true that we make time for what is most important to us? As sad as it may sound, it actually is a legitimate consideration if you examine it carefully. Why should you waste your time doing something that is not important to you?

If you cannot grasp the importance of having an effective exercise routine in your life, it is a waste of your time. From personal experience, I can assure you that where there is a lack in enjoyment or personal benefit, the lack of commitment will soon follow. There is a big difference in doing something because you are required to do it, and doing something because you want to do it. Imagine a scenario in which you are exercising because you want to. Imagine being able to say that you choose to exercise because of the benefits you enjoy from it. It is at this point that you must escape your imagination. Shall we bring your imagination into reality?

Exercising with Purpose is a workbook designed to help you establish a supportive environment in which you can succeed at your fitness goals, and get real results. After all, if you are going to put time and energy into something, you should be afforded a return on your investment. This workbook is for the individual who is "motivated" to take the necessary steps to improve their physicality and performance, by taking the time to develop a program that works for them. My goal is to help you capitalize on the spark of interest and motivation that you have in your personal fitness. Together, we will develop that spark into a consistent flame of growth and development. Every flame starts with a spark, but the tricky part is learning how to keep that flame lit.

If you are looking for a book overloaded with statistics and a solution to all of your problems, you should close this book. This workbook requires you to take ownership of your health. If you are too busy to make a lifestyle change for improving your health, your reading is done on this page. As the reader, you should know that the results you seek require dedication, commitment, and focus. If you are ready to take the necessary steps to accomplish your goals, I invite you to proceed to the next page.

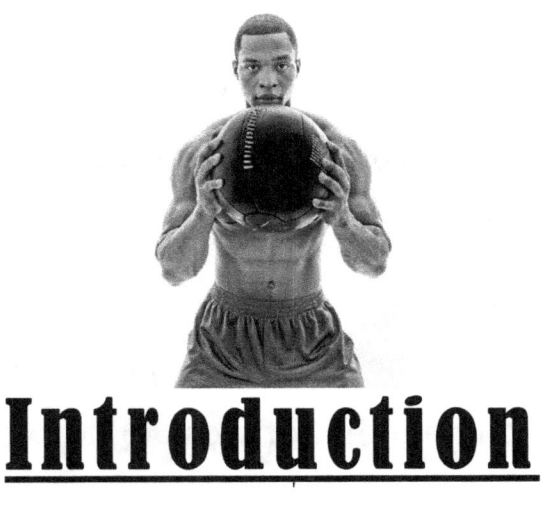

Introduction

When I think back to the initial spark of interest I had in improving my physical condition, I was only 12 years old, curious and driven by my imagination. My childhood was a bit different from the average 12 year old. My family lived a more simple life than most. I remember the times when I climbed trees, ran up and down hills, and explored the capabilities of my body. I was fairly strong before I knew what it meant to exercise. When my older brother played football for our high school, he sparked my interest in becoming stronger and fit. When I knew my brother played football, I wanted to learn more about the sport. One day I was watching a football game on the television. I was so amazed to see how the players controlled their movements on the field; I wanted to be able to mimic them in every way. After that day, I began running and did pushups daily to maintain a high fitness level, and then I finally stepped into my high school. My older brother always talked about how much he could bench press, and how fast he could run. You can imagine how excited I was when I finally discovered this place where one could spend time improving their appearance and performance. This place was called a "Weight Room" in my high school. Most kids spent time in the gymnasium but I preferred to be in the weight room. I wanted to get started early and I felt like I had a lot of work to do. It was at this point that I made a commitment to myself. I made a stern commitment to improve my health and fitness continually, until it was no longer possible.

What excited me most about the weight room was that I had the option of how much I wanted to improve my endurance, strength, and power. I was 14 years old and a freshman in high school when I started weight training with the football and basketball teams. The team players were huge, and they were lifting weight that was twice the amount of my body. I was shocked and impressed to see how strong, powerful, and fast the players were. The football team became my competition, and sparked my interest in physical fitness even more. I had a natural advantage, as my family lived a simple life for many years. My brothers and I all carried firewood, chopped wood, and worked with my father over the summer; my father was a carpenter. With this type of experience, I had a good understanding of what it meant to move and manipulate weight with my strength. When I began lifting weights in the weight room, I learned how to use this internal awareness of my strength to excel in the physical arena. I had a unique insight into fitness at a young age. After two years of lifting weights, I became curious about the meaning of total fitness. From then on, I knew the body was capable of so much more than anyone had imagined previously.

I maintained my interest in fitness as I grew older. As I reached puberty, I saw more muscle develop in the areas I had been working on so diligently, and I began to appreciate my physique much more. After getting a work permit, I started working at a local fast food restaurant. At the time, I did not know much about nutrition. I just knew that I needed to eat when I was hungry. After a few months of working behind the scenes, I learned that fast food was not the way to go. I was sickened by deep fried and fattening foods. As I worked daily in a fast food environment, I learned that I had to make some healthier choices about what I ate. I had to do what I could to maintain my health and fitness while being in an unhealthy environment. I began eating more vegetables, fruits, and lean meats. Unfortunately, I noticed the people around me were not conscious of maintaining their health. At my job, I realized people thought I was an athlete, or trying out for "the team" because I was into fitness. I began to wonder why an individual would think the idea of improving the body in a particular way was meant for certain people.

I graduated high school and joined the U.S. Navy when I was 17 years old. When I arrived at Navy bootcamp in 2001, I quickly learned what calisthenics were, and the benefits. Bootcamp was an experience like no other. Nothing compares to being sleep deprived constantly, and waking up at 4am in the morning to exercise. Nevertheless, I was in great shape afterwards. After leaving boot camp, I was introduced to the "weight room" again on a Navy school base. On the Navy base it was called a "gym". I began to refocus my mind on developing my body; using calisthenics, cardio, and weights. The physical changes that the body went through under controlled stress really kept my attention on fitness. I was captivated each time I achieved the results I wanted. During this period of my life, I began to research the human body and the effects of exercise, and I started to experiment with different forms of exercise. I learned that the human body is an amazing entity.

While serving in the U.S. Navy, I was excited about seeing different parts of the world, and seeing different body types and shapes. As I arrived on foreign lands, I was surprised to see that the idea of being sedentary was ok. I traveled to different parts of the world while serving in the U.S. Navy, such as Spain, Italy, Turkey, and Dubai. To my surprise, the attitudes about maintaining ones health were all the same. It was at this point when I learned that many people believed that health could be a consideration and not a priority. Many thoughts about maintaining fitness standards began to swirl in my head. Why would one choose not to maintain personal fitness standards throughout their life? When an individual chose to be sedentary, it was difficult for me to understand. I enjoyed having the ability to run, jump, and play sports, not to mention the good feeling it gave me when people commented on my physique.

Unknowingly, I had my first personal training experience during the year of 2001 in the U.S. Navy. One of my fellow sailors asked me to help him get in shape. My friend started having trouble fitting into his uniforms that once fit him so elegantly. I was sure that wearing clothes that did not fit was uncomfortable. He asked for my help after seeing my dedication to my personal fitness. I did not know what we were going to do exactly, I just told him to come to the gym with me, and we exercised together. I applied everything I read, researched, and learned. We ran and practiced weight training for three months. At the conclusion of those three months, his uniforms were too big, and his confidence radiated from within. I was so proud of him, and it brought me so much joy to see him work so hard for something he wanted so badly. I congratulated him, and encouraged him to stay on this path to maintain his fitness. Sadly, a few months later I saw him blow up like a balloon again. Needless to say, I was disappointed and saddened that he would give up months of hard work and dedication. Throughout my Navy experience, I trained more people, helped them get in shape, and watched them throw their hard work away just like my friend. Instead of being upset and giving up on everyone, I began to understand that everyone has different motivations for staying fit and that is something I cannot change. However, this did not exempt them from heart disease, diabetes, and other chronic health conditions stemming from living an unhealthy lifestyle. I soon left the navy and pursued my real passion. I wanted to change lives and save lives. Eventually, I began working as a personal trainer at a local gym in Jacksonville, Florida. I really enjoyed it, as it was a very rewarding occupation. I was back in the gym, doing what I loved best, staying fit and helping others become fit. Unfortunately, I started to get an old feeling again. I began to feel a sense of boredom, and suddenly I was overcome with the need to attend to those who really needed my services. From my repeated experiences, I learned that a commitment to fitness had to be a personal decision.

Health and Fitness hit home for me when a tragic event made its way into my life. Unfortunately, over time I would soon discover my mother would be diagnosed with Congestive Heart Failure. On September 10, 2006, I went home as I normally would, to spend time with my family. I spent the last few hours of my visit watching television with my mother. I could hear her heavy breathing as she fell asleep during a television show. I left Georgia that night, and drove home to my apartment in Jacksonville, Florida. On September 11, 2006, my sister called me to inform me that our mother died from a massive heart attack. I had a hard time accepting this news, and could not find my passion to keep working. After a few weeks I began working productively again. Suddenly, health and fitness had a new meaning. I began a personal crusade against chronic and preventable health conditions, as I had a sudden realization of the number of deaths caused by the lack of health education and unhealthy living.

After my mother's death, my training style became more educational. I began to put my focus on the individual who had a true desire to be healthy and fit. I remembered the days of helping someone attain their goals, only to watch them throw it away; that was my past. I found my passion again but still I felt there was something missing. I wanted to teach a person exercise techniques that would help prevent chronic health conditions and help them maintain fitness standards they set for themselves. There had to be an effective way to send out a warning that everyone could see and hear. There were plenty of commercials, compact discs, and books that show you how to "get ripped", "gain muscle mass", and "get a six pack". Unfortunately, exercising for superficial gain often leaves one empty handed and unmotivated to continue. I decided to throw a big wrench into this useless cycle. I designed this workbook to assist an individual in understanding their personal health and fitness. Keeping that in mind, I created this manual to help individuals protect their health and save lives. I am about to take you on a unique journey of getting fit, staying fit, and learning how to enjoy it. I am going to teach you a secret that will change your life, if you are ready to be a student.

In our society today, there are a large number of individuals who are sedentary. It is now a common event to hear of a friend, or family member developing a chronic health condition when living a sedentary and unhealthy lifestyle. Unfortunately, we are not connecting the dots, when it comes to maintaining a healthy lifestyle. Sadly, we accept the many reasons and excuses a person may have to ignore the status of their health. If we are to pursue our dreams in life, and provide a secure environment for our families, we cannot afford to look at maintaining good health as an option. When you dream of attaining a certain lifestyle through hard work, are you carrying around an oxygen tank to breathe? When you dreamed about having a family, were you having trouble with your weight? I emphasize this because we are "happy and healthy" in our dreams. I hope it is a clear signal to you, the reader of this book that health contributes to happiness tremendously.

From a young age, we learn how to eat unhealthy foods, and have been trained to seek out what tastes good instead of what is actually good for the body. Look around you; the number of obese children continues to increase daily. Can you see it? According to the Center for Disease Control, obesity among children has tripled in the last 30 years. Look at your neighbor. If they had to run 200 meters (1/4 mile), do you think they could complete this task without panting and gasping for air? Unfortunately, most people cannot participate in an intense activity for more than 1 minute without having shortness of breath. If you asked most of your friends and family to tell you the digestive process, and give you details on the anatomy of the human body, most of them would probably have little information to give you. If you asked them to name the cast members in their favorite television show, or all the members of their favorite sports team, they could tell you with ease and confidence, all the names, and maybe more details. Sadly, many individuals are clueless about their bodies, the very thing that allows us to experience the highest quality of life possible. What is more disturbing is that most of these individuals are our children, who we are counting on to be the future leaders of tomorrow. How can a child achieve their full potential without their health? What I am pointing out is the lack in knowledge of the human body and its functions. What is more disturbing is the lack in the desire to learn about the human body. We would take hours to learn about our favorite car before we take minutes to see what makes our own engine run. We seem to be invincible until our bodies break down, and then we pity ourselves as if we were cursed. There is something wrong with this scenario. Do you agree?

In my personal opinion, lack of knowledge about the human body stems from many events that happen throughout our lives. I am sure you will agree. Unfortunately, we are forced to learn most of the information about our bodies when we have zero interest in the subject. How much interest did you have in human anatomy when you were a child or adolescent? We are human beings and we like to spend our time doing things that are fun, enjoyable, that will not bore us to sleep. Our lives take us through a unique cycle. When we are younger, life is fun and adventurous. We play sports, play with friends, and have active vacations. Sadly, as we grow older and take on more responsibilities, the world of adult life almost forces us to dismiss the idea of being active and physically fit. Work and family life become more demanding, and consume the little free time we have. As our lives continue, we are forced to multitask, and make less time for our health. Are you seeing what I am seeing? Our lifestyle has a large impact on our health.

Lack of interest is another major issue, and can stem from many events in our lives as well. The idea of being fit has changed over the years. If you were to seek information on getting fit, most people would tell you to go to a gym. We all know exactly where to go. If you took a poll, you would find most people want to be healthy, fit, attractive, and energetic. However, you would find most of them do not want to walk on a treadmill for hours, or lift weights, and put themselves in pain. Do you see this broken cycle? People like you want to take part in fun activities that stimulate your mind and senses. You were not created to stand still you were created to move. Although, you will have to condition yourself and get fit before you can get involved in some intense and fun activities. Would you like to know what you are capable of? So, enough chitchat, let's get moving.

My goal with this interactive workbook is to help you establish fitness goals, design a sustainable plan that works for you, get you focused on what is really important, and have a lot of fun during the process. Stop being frustrated and do what works best for you. It is a simple formula; do what works for you.

You are about to take a journey that will require you to take specific steps for successful completion. Always remember that a journey starts with the first step. The steps in this workbook are designed to help you find the most success in your journey to health and fitness. Take your time! Slow and steady may not win every race, but it wins this one.

Notes

Step 1

Finding Purpose

Logically, you should understand the underlying principal and a short history of fitness before you begin your unique journey. You must now allow your memory to travel back in time, before technology, when man possessed the necessary physical skills for survival.

Naturally, the more primitive man was required to have the physical skills to hunt and gather food for survival. Hunting did not mean getting the shotgun and shooting what was in your back yard. It meant miles of traveling and tracking to find your next meal. Unfortunately, the work was not complete when you acquired your food. You then had to carry your food the same miles you traveled from home to feed the village. When you arrived at home, you participated in festivities to celebrate the hunt. Could you imagine working this hard for one of your meals? A high fitness level was necessary to survive during this time, and the daily routine naturally kept individuals physically fit. There was no need to schedule a separate time for the purpose of improving one's physical fitness.

The sedentary lifestyle began with the establishment of more complex civilizations. Eventually, human civilization learned how to farm, and did not need to hunt and gather our food as much. Although these changes evolved differently throughout the world, the fact remains that we became more sedentary over time.

With civilization came the birth of ancient fitness forms such as Martial Arts and Yoga. These were the first notable forms of organized physical fitness. Martial Arts and Yoga emphasized keeping the mind and body in a proper working condition through physical and mental discipline. Though the specific art forms and practices had a specific purpose, one could not achieve growth without being physically fit in some manner.

Who would doubt that the Greek Civilization contributed tremendously to the idea of an individual maintaining an admirable physique? The Greek Civilization gave birth to the Olympic Games. The Olympic Games brought a large focus on having a training regimen to achieve a certain fitness level. One can only imagine how a prospective Olympic Athlete qualified to participate in the Olympic Games. Nevertheless, an Olympic Athlete obviously trained their bodies to perfect their skills for intense competition. Although many different games took place in various countries, the Olympic Games still are the largest event where top athletes around the world compete.

The military also provided a basis of fitness. The military required a soldier to be "fit for duty". The soldier, sailor, or marine needed to be fit for duty to carry out his required purpose in the military branch he served. Specific levels of fitness, such as running, jumping, climbing, and swimming were all requirements for a soldier, sailor, or marine to carry out his duties effectively. An unfit member of the military would be a liability to all those in his unit as they are required to function as one unit.

After the Olympic Games, we were introduced to other organized games such as Lacrosse, Soccer, Baseball, Football, Basketball, and Hockey. These were the hallmarks of team sports; which have flourished since the late 1800's. As sports and fitness became more popular, the Gymnasium was born. The introduction of the Gymnasium in schools was for the accommodation of individual games and team sports. The YMCA was one of the pioneers in fitness; focusing on the importance of having a "healthy body" as one of their core values. The YMCA led the way in creating gymnasiums all over the United States in the late 1800's. By the late 1900's, physical education was a requirement in most schools; combating the rising obesity problem in the world. Eventually, Health Clubs stemmed from the idea of having physical education incorporated into the school system. Health Clubs provided a great environment for people interested in physical fitness. Interested parties could continue their fitness efforts beyond the gymnasium into adulthood.

Over the years, one will notice how the kinesthetic awareness in the human society has drastically declined. Kinesthetic Awareness, in simple terms, can be defined as the awareness of the body. Have you ever been in a situation in which you were required to manipulate your body to complete a task? Yet, you hesitated because you were simply unsure of your abilities. Have you ever been in a situation in which you completed an arduous physical task without thinking twice about it? Maybe you can dunk a basketball or you can perform a somersault. Have you ever tried to throw a piece of paper in the trashcan from far away? Yes, even the smallest tasks in your life require that you have a certain awareness of the body. An individual becomes more confident in their abilities as they develop their kinesthetic awareness. Naturally, individuals who participate in sports activities and perform other physical activities on a routine basis have a greater sense of what their body is capable of. As we become more sedentary, our awareness starts to decline, and we become unaware of our physical abilities. Fortunately, we have the power to make improvements in our physical abilities any time we wish. Would it not feel good to have confidence in the abilities of your body once again? What are you waiting for?

There are so many changes that have led up to the world in which we live today. We provide for our families with jobs that require little to no physical exertion, we are plugged into the Internet, and our ears are glued to our cell phones. We are not required to hunt and gather our food anymore, and we seek instant results for the efforts we put into any task. Unfortunately, the majority of the world's population is not participating in any Olympic Games or participating in professional sports. Most of us are not fighting in wars around the world, and physical education is now being taken out of schools. We are now teaching our children that being physically fit is less important than maintaining good grades in school. Our lifestyles are so busy that we prefer to eat fast food instead of more nutritious foods. We are well aware of the consequences of living an unhealthy lifestyle. Yet, a large portion of the population makes the unhealthy choice, so that we may keep up with our fast paced society. The examples set for the young children in the world are more troubling. Unfortunately, after the amazing history of fitness, here we are, with no particular reason to maintain or care about our fitness. Our physical education and fitness now relies on health clubs, exercise television, and magazines; which are all driven by money and product selling. What are we to do? Great Question!

When you think of what it means exercise in today's society, images of people participating in physical activities start to circulate through your mind in different ways. Some of the images are of people in the gym lifting weights, or participating in group exercise classes. Some people are outside for their routine jog. Some people are at home using latest and greatest exercise video. We are well oriented with the different options available to us.

Although there are many people who choose not to live an active and healthy lifestyle, there are many who choose life. The decision to maintain fitness and health is one of the most important decisions a person can make. When a person decides to maintain their health, he/she has established in their minds that there is a reason for them to ensure that they contribute to their personal longevity. In my professional opinion, there are four major reasons why people exercise: superficial gain, long-term benefits, performance enhancing, and acts of desperation.

Superficial Gain

Who would not want to improve their physical appearance? Would you like a nice tone and shape for your body? Obviously, most people have some desire to make improvements to their body. Since the dawn of civilization, we have known that having a strong body was the right way to enhance our appearance. At some point in our lives, we all have pursued the act of enhancing our physique. It may have been flat stomach we desired. Maybe we wanted our legs more toned and muscular. Maybe we wanted to add more muscle in the chest and arm areas. Whatever it was, it is likely that at some point of our lives we thought about enhancing our physique.

Over time, the reasons for wanting to enhance our physique may have varied. Was there someone we wanted to impress? Was there a special event coming up? No matter the reason, we were focused on getting in shape, and we had a deadline in which the task needed to be completed. We thought about it daily, and practiced with intensity. Nothing could get in the way of us getting in shape. If an obstacle did come up, still we found a way to get the job done.

Enhancing your appearance is a great way to build confidence. The desire to enhance your appearance is not a bad thing. It is the first impression people get from you. Why not make it a good one? First impressions are very important in all aspects of our life. Are you preparing for an interview? Are you going on a first date with someone? Are you a salesman or saleswoman? No matter the scenario, we will all eventually have the event of a first impression appear in our lives. What will you impress upon the person that you encounter?

Long-Term Benefits

For some of us, it does not take much to get moving. We did our research, and understand the long-term benefits of regular exercise and healthy living. We know that lack of physical activity increases our risk of chronic diseases, and may have other disastrous effects on our lives. We may have a relative that suffers from a condition that could have been avoided by practicing a healthy lifestyle. Some of us are parents who would like to ensure we are healthy enough to support and watch our kids prosper. Many people could not bear the thought of suffering from something which was entirely preventable, and caused only by their personal behavior. Along the same lines, we do not want to be in a position in which we are forced to deal with a preventable health issue. In our daily lives we are reminded of the impact a healthy lifestyle has on our lives and our health. So why wait to preserve your health? After all, we all want to live fulfilling lives.

According to the American Heart Association, physical activity reduces risks of heart disease, improves cholesterol levels, helps manage stress, helps to slow down and prevent chronic illnesses, and much more. The American Heart Association also points out the fact that the number of sedentary jobs has increased 83% since 1953. That statistic means that most of today's employees are sedentary for the majority of their day. The American Heart Association also points out that it costs an employer up to $2500 per year in medical costs and sick days per year. If I were an employer, I would be selective about who I would hire. Would you not do the same?

Performance Enhancing

Some us like to study the effects of exercise in relation to the body's capabilities. We play sports regularly, have a job that is very physical, or maybe we like to experiment. Either way, enhancing your performance is something very personal. We can train ourselves to run faster, jump higher, increase our endurance, improve strength, and improve our skills to become a better competitor. Performance enhancing sparks from those who want to achieve specific performance goals by improving their performance in certain areas. Within ourselves, each and every one of us has the most powerful tool we need to succeed. That tool is the desire to set goals for yourself and the willpower to attain those goals.

Among most health professionals, it is known widely that exercise increases oxygen flow to the brain, allowing the individual to carry out cognitive functions better and remain more alert. Exercise does more than train the body; it trains the brain. By physically training your body, you increase the consistency in your performance by building muscle memory. Muscle memory (motor learning) means that after repeating a specific movement consistently, the muscle develops the ability to perform the movement unconsciously. A good example of muscle memory is riding a bike. What do your muscles remember?

Every individual can benefit from improved performance. Examine the tasks you perform daily. What could you do to enhance your performance? How much time could it save you? How much money could it save you? In what way will it increase your production? Enhance your performance and reap the benefits of having more energy, stamina, and production.

Acts of Desperation

Acts of desperation can cause us to exercise; however, an act of desperation is not necessarily a good building block. It usually causes us to act out of fear, and make irrational decisions. As a result, our reason for exercise becomes induced by fear.

Take this scenario for example:

Danny was very active when he was younger. He played sports his entire life, until he acquired his college degree and a demanding job. He started putting in long hours at work, and eventually he got married. After marriage, Danny started a family, and lost track of his exercise routine. After turning 35, he was informed by his doctor that his cholesterol levels were too high. Danny wanted to make better decisions to be healthy, so that he could protect his health. Without questioning, he understood and agreed with the benefits he could receive from exercising, but did not know how or where to start. He was active earlier in his life. How hard could it be? Impatiently, Danny wanted to improve his performance, physique, and receive the long-term benefits. He did not take the time to condition, nor did he understand his limitations. Yet, in desperation he pushed too hard in his exercise program, and then became discouraged and disinterested quickly. Without taking the time to understand his situation and relying on ego, Danny set himself up for failure. He never tried to exercise again, and decided that exercising simply was not for him.

Most people can avoid the consequences of being sedentary by maintaining a consistent exercise routine. With that being said, the increase of chronic health conditions associated with a sedentary lifestyle should not be a surprise. Exercising moderately on a daily basis can prevent many chronic health conditions. After you have put your health as a priority, acquire assistance from a qualified fitness professional, who could develop an individualized exercise plan for you.

What is your story?

One of the most important decisions you can make in your life is the decision to maintain your health. What is your purpose for exercising? Do you exercise for superficial gain? Are you exercising for the long-term benefits? Does exercise give you mental clarity? Are you exercising to enhance your performance? Have you started exercising out of desperation? It is possible that you exercise for multiple reasons. We will all develop a different purpose to exercise throughout life as we embark on our personal journey to maintain our personal health. Take a look at some of these scenarios below. Could your situation have the same outcome?

Scenario 1: If you are a younger adult, you have plenty of exciting things to do with your spare time. When you get the opportunity, you try to enjoy the little freedom you are allowed. The last thing on your mind would be getting into the gym, and putting yourself through a hard workout. Unconsciously, you start to look around at the students in your class and on the school grounds, and you start seeing the harsh reality of the health problems that plague the young generation. You start noticing that many of the people you know are not active, and they do not want to be. You have a choice to make. You could remain sedentary like most people, or you could take ownership of your health. You decide to be more health conscious, and take ownership of your health. Although it is not a big issue at the moment, you know it will pay off later in life. You do not want to be unhealthy or out of shape, and you choose to make healthier decisions. After taking some time to learn about health and fitness, you find an exercise routine that matches your lifestyle and fits your personality. It was not as difficult as you thought it was. After a few months you are looking better, feel better, and wonder why you did not start earlier.

Scenario 2: You just made it to college, and started a new life on your own. Much of your normal routine has changed dramatically. Your life is much busier now, as you have become a full time student. You study constantly, and your feet are always on the move. Every week you have tests, and, whenever you get a chance, you hang out with friends or find peace. Exercising is not on the menu or agenda. You would like to exercise to enjoy the benefits. Unfortunately, you feel you do not have the time or motivation. As you scan the campus, you see everyone starting to put on their "freshman 30" and some putting on the "freshmen 50". Unable to see yourself carrying around an extra 50lbs in addition to your books, you set priorities, and get a workout partner to keep you motivated and accountable. After a few weeks of consistency, you see the benefits and love the way you look.

Scenario 3: You just celebrated your 40th birthday. In your younger years, you exercised for appearance and strength. After settling down, you shifted your focus to maintaining health and longevity. Your kids are growing fast, and your family needs you to be able to provide for them. Your family depends on you too much for a health issue to become part of the family equation. Over the years, you began to see the disastrous effects from heavy lifting and not working out. You look around at many of your friends and they look terrible. With your conscious eating at you, you decide to do what is best for your body and the family. You develop an exercise routine that keeps your heart healthy, keeps you flexible, keeps you strong, and clears your mind. After a few months you look better, and feel better. You feel confident knowing that you are protecting your ability to provide for your family.

Scenario 4: You made it to the 4th quarter of life, and you are still going strong. You never really thought about exercising, but knew it was a good thing for you at any age. You worked long and hard throughout your entire life to get to this point, and you are finally here; in the retirement age. You want to retire, but also know you want to retire healthy. Now that you have more time, you focus on your health and fitness, to increase your longevity. You hire a personal trainer to show you age appropriate exercises, and begin your personal journey. After exercising and eating well for a few months, you realize how important it is to engage the body in the discipline of physical fitness. After some time, you also realize how exercise contributes to a better functioning mind and body. You made a decision to age gracefully.

Summary

Most of the things we practice with consistency and discipline in our lives actually have strong purpose enforcing them. We work because we need to make money and support our families. We choose to travel many hours because of the emotional reward that comes from visiting close friends and family members. We take our pets to the vet because they have been so loyal to us in the past, and they deserve all the care and attention we can give them. Although these events all take precious time away from our lives, they give us great personal satisfaction, and are all contributing to give us the quality of life we are seeking.

There is nothing different about having a purpose to exercise. In fact, there is nothing different about having a purpose to do anything in your life. Everything you are pursuing and practicing currently in your life is majorly what you choose to do. Making progress is all about setting priorities, and defining what and how you want your quality of life to be.

When you think of your purpose of exercising, it should have an afterthought. Start with this sentence, "I am doing this because…" now finish the sentence. Unfortunately, for most of us there usually is not an afterthought. For many of us, exercising is just a way to improve appearance and nothing more. When you think of your purpose for exercising, imagine the benefit you would gain from reaching a certain goal, and continue elaborating on the benefits more. How do you attain the most benefit from exercising? Think of something that involves the people you love. Think of something you could do for yourself that benefits the people you love. You may want to think of a personal experience; I did. For me, that personal experience for me was my mother's death. After my mother's death, I no longer needed a reason to maintain my health and fitness.

I am about to get you set on the right track, so that you may move forward in your journey. The first project is designed for you to find a purpose and/or reason for exercising. It is simple, fill in the blanks honestly, and the rest will take care of itself. If you are honest and true with your answers, you will begin to build your steps to success. Complete this exercise like your life depended on it, because it does.

Exercise: What is my purpose?

Upon completion of this exercise, you will develop a defined purpose for pursuing a personal fitness standard. Complete each sentence based on what area it applies to in your life. Read the questions carefully, as they will appear similar but are different.

A. In my personal opinion, exercise is good for the body

because_____

_____

_____

B. Exercising will help me _____

  better.

C. My family depends on my health in this way:

_____

_____

_____

_____

D. What I value the most in terms of health is?

_____

_____

_____

_____

_____

_____

_____

E. My health affects my ability to work or study in this way:

_____

_____

F. My health could possibly be a personal burden if:

_____

_____

_____

G. Taking ownership of my health would allow me to

_____

_____

H. In 25 years I would like my health to be

_____ because

_____

_____

A Strong Foundation

At this point, you should have a good idea of your purpose and/or reason for exercising. You should have also identified your wants and needs that relate to fitness. Without sufficient health, your world comes to a complete stop.

It is quite clear that our health and fitness affects us in almost every area of our lives. While answering the previous questions, you may have noticed that they related to all areas of your life: family, friends, health, job, and your future. Health must be present at all times during your life, in order for you to achieve your full potential in all the areas of your life. We would all like to live long lives, but we do not want to live our lives with a chronic illness, or in a state of constant suffering. Unfortunately, an unhealthy lifestyle is the path many individuals are following. Take a look around your daily environment; obviously, you will notice many people are having trouble maintaining their health. There are more cases of childhood obesity, more people are being diagnosed with diabetes, and the cases of heart disease are on the rise. Without a purpose for maintaining health, practicing a healthy lifestyle is simply a waste of time. It is essential for you to find a purpose for exercising. When you develop a strong and definite purpose to accomplish a task, you will strive to be the best you can be in that area. It is that simple! How great does it feel to know that you just took the time to evaluate how health plays an important role in your lifestyle? You now know your purpose for exercising. Your purpose is the reason why you will choose to be active every day. Notice, your answers to the previous questions had nothing to do with more muscle tone, increased muscle size, or losing weight. Superficial goals are important, however, there are greater benefits than physical gains. You chose those answers because you recognize those greater benefits. You made those choices because you want to live a healthy lifestyle, and be the best you can. Your purpose is something you believe strongly, and are motivated to accomplish. Having a strong and definite purpose takes the hassle out of the process itself. All the events we engage in daily have a process for completion. The motivations we have for events are what make them different.

Notes

Take some time to reflect on what you have learned about yourself from this chapter. Write down the things most important to you in your life, and what they mean to you. What is your reason for waking up every morning? Think about these important parts of your life and use them for motivation when you exercise.

_____

_____

_____

_____

_____

_____

_____

_____

_____

Step 2

Setting Goals

The word "goal", relating to achievements, is defined as "the object of a person's ambition or effort; an aim or desired result". A goal must be clear, concise, and measurable. I want to clarify what a goal is by saying it is something you can see, feel, touch, and accomplish in a certain time frame. Ultimately, your goal must be realistic but challenging. A challenging goal should be out of reach, but within your grasp. The goal should make you push yourself a bit harder to accomplish it. A good goal will allow you to grow, gain confidence in your abilities, and develop character. In any case, when you specify your goals, you give yourself a chance to pursue the goal effectively.

Take a look at the following examples:

Unspecified: I want to lose my gut

Specified: I am in a size 10 now and I want to get into a size 6 in 3 months. Today it is July 1st and I want to accomplish this by the end of September.

Unspecified: I want to run my mile in a faster time.
Specified: My current mile time is 10 minutes and I want to run a mile in 8 minutes after a month of training. Today it is September 15th. I want to bring my time down by October 15th.

Notice, the unspecified goals do not have numbers or time limits. Establishing diverse and undefined goals will most likely lead you down an undefined path but never to your "goal". Goals without deadlines and numbers to improve upon can waste valuable time. By giving yourself a marker or an ending, you have something to pursue; work smarter not harder. Defining your goal is very simple process. You keep the process simple by developing goals with specific numbers, times, and date. Success will come if you COMMIT TO THE NUMBERS AND YOUR GOAL. Commit as Ramu did when we established his personal goals.

I met Ramu Akula during an early morning as I was walking out of a fitness center. He was waiting for me to finish a training session, and wanted to talk with me about developing a fitness plan. Ramu explained he was tired of being overweight and unhealthy. He was diagnosed with diabetes, he was a new father, providing for his family, and he did not know how to maintain his fitness. Ramu was concerned about his longevity and quality of life. He had no problem admitting that he needed help.

Ramu had a very common issue. He knew little about exercising, and had the tremendous responsibility of being the sole provider of his family, a father, and a husband. Ramu definitely had a purpose for getting in shape, but did not have clear goals, nor did he have the knowledge to pursue the results he wanted.

After Ramu and I sat down for an interview, we established specific goals, and prepared to make progress. As I evaluated him, I could see that he was very much out of shape after living a sedentary lifestyle. Although this was true, his current physical condition did not slow him down. After a few weeks of conditioning, Ramu was eager to pursue his goals. At the time of our interview, he weighed 190lbs and had a 36-inch waist. His goal was to lose 20lbs and 4 inches in 6 months.

After Ramu established his goals, he was able to establish a target. He now had something to pursue, and he did that exactly, with intense determination and focus. Ramu listened intently as I explained to him the purpose of specific exercises, why it was important to avoid certain foods, and why it was more important for him to exercise when he was not with me. He battled fiercely with the changes he had to make. In the end, Ramu changed his lifestyle, improved his health, and regained his confidence by asking for help and committing to his goals. Ramu even made changes to his traditional eating, from the culture of India. The transition was hard for him, but he was willing to fight for his health. While pursuing his personal goals, Ramu made such an impression on his fellow employees, that he influenced them to change their lives as well.

We can change our circumstances at the time of our choosing. In many cases, do not have to wait for the right time, and when we do, it is because we are procrastinating. The power to make change is in your hands. Gain insight from the experience Ramu had. He knew nothing about exercising, and was willing to learn what was necessary to maintain his health. Ramu continues to exercise daily, looks better, feels better, and is controlling his diabetes effortlessly. In three months, Ramu lost 20lbs and lost 4 inches in his waist. He just wanted to win bad enough. Take ownership of your health and stop settling. Taking ownership of your health is one decision you will never regret.

Although accomplishing your goal is a great feat, it does not mean your work is finished. When you establish a goal, you must understand that your goals are subject to change, and will change. You may lose interest in your goal, or your initial purpose could change. Maybe you will get tired of the routine you developed? Did your schedule change? Is there a new member of the family? I could go on and on. Accept the fact that your goals are subject to change. It is just the way life is, and change is okay. If you become bored with your current exercise routine, or you become disinterested in your current goal, it is okay. Losing momentum when you are trying to go up a hill is natural, and you are allowed to be human. DO NOT GIVE UP! When the battle gets tough, dig in deeper and push harder. Make all of your efforts count, by keeping a close eye on your progress. Re-evaluate your goals and your interest level monthly. Even if you have been attempting to accomplish a goal for six years, it is okay to lose interest, and it does not mean you are going to lose everything you worked for if you change your goals.

Your goals and your purpose are two different animals. Your purpose can be measured on a much larger scale than your goal. Think of your purpose as the path you choose to take. Your goals are the roads you can build to go anywhere you want within your path. As long as you have a path, you can build roads to take you wherever you want to go. With that being said, without a path, you cannot go anywhere. Your goals give you landmarks to look for during your journey, and they reward you as you reach checkpoints during the journey. The journey could be long, which is why being rewarded at times is so important. Maintaining your interest in something for an extended period can be challenging, if a personal reward is absent.

How do we make our goals personal? From my personal experience, I have notice there are three types of goals that keep me moving. I divide these goals in relation to performance, physical, and ego.

Exercise: Establishing Specific Goals

Upon completing this exercise, you will have established your specific short term, intermediate, and long term goals. Remember, the goals must be specific with times, dates, and numbers. Write down the goals that provide you with an intense desire for their completion. Within each time period, you will write down a goal that measures your performance, physical changes, and satisfies and/or challenges your ego. Think about goals on a personal level, and make them relate to your purpose. Also, remember your goals can and will change in the future.

Performance goals will challenge you in terms of your fitness. A performance goal could be pushups, lifting weights, running a mile, or being active in a certain sport. **Physical** goals will challenge you in terms of your physical appearance. A physical goal can relate to weight, inches, and muscle tone. Goals that challenge your **ego** will take you out of your comfort zone, and allow you to feel a sense of pride after completing a personal goal. A goal associated with your ego, will pertain to you pursuing something you made a commitment to do when you were in shape. Think of a goal associated with your ego as a celebration of your fitness achievements.

Example of Month Goal:

Goal Dates:

February 16 – March 16

Physical:

I want to lose 2 inches in one month

Performance:

I want to run a mile in 8 minutes

Ego- Oriented:

I will take those dance lessons I have been thinking about.

You will need specific goals, accompanied by your workout routine, to make progress. In any case, establishing specific goals will prevent you from exercising in vain, and ensure that you will always work hard to achieve your goals. There is nothing worse than going to the gym just because you know you need to; how boring! Feel free to write down more than one goal for each category. Although options are great, only pursue one goal from each category to avoid losing focus, and maintaining your consistency in progress.

Short Term Goals: Something you feel can be obtained within 1-3 months.

Performance Goals:

_____

_____

_____

Physical Goals:

_____

_____

_____

Ego-oriented Goals:

_____

_____

_____

Intermediate Goals: A goal you can meet within 3-6 months

Performance Goals:

_____

_____

_____

Physical Goals:

_____

_____

_____

Ego-oriented Goals:

_____

_____

_____

Long Term Goals: A goal you can meet within 6-12 months.

Performance Goals:

_____

_____

_____

Physical Goals:

_____

_____

_____

Ego-oriented Goals:

_____

_____

_____

You want it? Then go after it!

At this point, you have a destination and a few items to pursue. You can now make progress. It is just that simple. You get your plan together, and you figure out a way to execute it in the most effective manner. Your purpose gave you a path, and now your goals are your roadmap. It would be unwise to start a journey without a map and a path. After you have established your short term, intermediate, and long term goals, there are only a few things left to do: take a photo, post your goals, tell your friends.

Post your goals and your photo in a place where you think deeply about your appearance. Photos will serve as a visual reminder of what you are fighting for, and what irritates you about your body, and will show the progress of your hard work.   Your friends will serve as a constant reminder and accountability to your commitments. Make your journey to success personal by finding a way to make it more exciting and interactive: scrapbook, weekly photo, or challenging a friend. When exercising, having a stimulus keeps you focused on the bull's-eye.

You are almost ready to go on your journey. You know your purpose and you have personal goals. Unfortunately, the journey is not just a walk in the park. You need to know what you are up against, and what challenges lie in your path. Educating yourself about what you want to accomplish will help you avoid unexpected obstacles along the way. Do not be so eager to change your world, you will be eaten alive before you can comprehend what is happening. Always start with baby steps. Education can be attained in the form of research, watching videos, using a qualified health or fitness professional, and understanding your personality and body. Attaining knowledge is where you put in the real work. As you read ahead, you will attain the knowledge necessary to accomplish your goals.

Notes

Step 3

Body Types

The body of each human being varies in size, shape, weight, and many other ways. If you turn on your television, turn the pages in your favorite magazine, or walk out your front door, it is highly unlikely that the first person we encounter will have a body type that matches our own. When you think of it this way, it becomes obvious that we all have different body types. These different body types will shape, build muscle, and retain fat in different ways. Understanding basic characteristics of different body types will give you tremendous insight into what you are able to accomplish physically. Knowledge of different body shapes is not new information, but it is often overlooked. In fact, William Sheldon PhD marked our basic understanding of body shapes in the 1940's. When we look at our neighbor, we are completely aware of the differences and similarities in our body structures. In fact, we see the differences and comparisons every day. Your best friend could be considered "skinny". Your boss could be considered "stocky". The information that differentiates our bodies is introduced to us visually on a daily basis. In other words, we are aware of the different shapes and know what category we fall in.

Unfortunately, when we want to start an exercise program, we easily forget about common differences in body structures. When we are out of shape, we automatically produce an image of what we would like to look like in our minds. The image may come from someone we saw on television, in a magazine, or someone in our neighborhood gym. Many times we overlook the complexity of these images. While the thought of achieving your desired shape can be invigorating, there are many thoughts to contemplate before we process an image of fitness or beauty.

What kind of body type do you have, and what type of maintenance should you perform on it? There are many different descriptions of body types. According to William Sheldon PhD, there are three major body types; ectomorph, mesomorph, and endomorph. In this manual, I will make the body types easy for you to remember, by using five distinct body shapes we can all relate to. The five body shapes I will use in this chapter are: V-shape, hourglass, apple, pear, and banana.

1) The "V-shape" is basically what it sounds like. The upper torso area is much wider than the narrow waist and hips.

2) The body with an "hourglass" shape is basically a body that has a narrow waist accompanied by a wider upper torso area and hips.

3) The "apple" body type has most of the body weight distributed in the middle of the body.

4) The "pear" body type has most of the body weight distributed in the lower body.

5) A banana shaped body is evenly proportionate from torso to hips.

Now that you are informed about the different body types, try to narrow down the one that resembles your shape the most. Take a look in the mirror and analyze your shape. You could possibly be a combination of two body types. Understanding the characteristics of your body type is very important. If you know specific characteristics of your body type, you can tackle the specific issues that your body type normally encounters. By understanding your body type, you will eliminate confusion, and then establish certain parameters in your goals and routines. Most of all, you will not formulate your goals based on a body type that does not match yours. Instead, you allow yourself to focus on your problem areas and take advantage of the natural strengths of your body.

I understand completely how easy it is to see something you like, and then get motivated to pursue that goal. During your journey, motivation is very important for achieving goals. Without motivation, achieving a goal becomes a bit challenging. Nevertheless, having proper motivation for your situation is what is most important. The majority of our desire to become physically fit stems from images we have come to admire. Analyze one of these images of what you think is "beauty" or "fit"; visualize it clearly in your mind. What kind of body type does this person have? Does that body type resemble yours in any way? How did that person achieve those results? Is it possible that the person achieved those results in an unhealthy fashion? Did they take supplements or skip meals; the truth is we will never know. If you know the person that you come to admire, ask them questions. At least you will know the truth of their efforts.

What should I do? Understanding your body type is one of the most important things you can do regarding your personal fitness. Think of the different models of cars in the world. Each one of them is built for a specific purpose, and requires a different type of maintenance. The maintenance you perform on a family van would not work on a sports car. Although some things are similar about the two vehicles, much more varies in their relation. The different body types of humans relate in the same manner. Different body types require different maintenance.

As you begin to age more, you will find that your body follows the same pattern. With time and age, changes in the body are a natural phenomenon. You may notice that an elderly person's appearance is significantly different from their pictures in their youth. Aging is a natural process that we all experience. Being aware of your body as it goes through the aging process, allows you to adapt to different situations when necessary. Over time, you may have to change your workouts to match the natural changes in your body. Awareness of natural changes in the body comes in handy when maintaining personal fitness.

Summary

When you understand the differences in body types, you will make informed decisions about the goals you choose to accomplish. As you conduct your own research about your body, you will find many facts that will help you discover the true nature of how it exists. Naturally, we are all curious about our body and how it functions. To gather a true understanding of your body, you must become a student of it. Everything you need to know about your body cannot be found in a book, it comes from personal insight and experience.

Notes

Step 4

Exercise Routine

I met Arman Moeini in the summer of 2007; yet, that day remains fresh in my mind. Arman walked into the front door of the studio I worked at with intimidation, and he did not have a particular interest in fitness. He was 14 years old, and at the heaviest weight he had been in his life. I knew he was not pleased with the way he looked. After talking with Arman, I knew he wanted to look and feel better about himself. He was not interested in the superficial gains, and wanted to be healthy for himself.

Arman was no stranger to exercise. In fact, he played football, was on the weightlifting team, and was on the school lacrosse team at the time. Although these were intense sports, Arman expressed that he did not have a definite interest in them. The fact that Arman played sports made the situation all the more frustrating; he was not a kid sitting on the couch. He kept himself active and was participating in team sports. The circumstances were there, but something seemed out of place. Nevertheless, he wanted to work hard at something and get the results he sought after. There was something that needed to change, and Arman was on a mission to find it.

A year went by, during which Arman and I met sporadically, and I did not know how long it would take him to find his motivation. In August 2008, Arman and I talked again about his goals, only this time he was focused. When I looked in his eyes, I knew that he was about to change his life. He had found what he needed within himself. Arman was about to start the 10th grade, and he was changing schools. I could see that he intended to act on the change he wanted to see within himself as we sat down and talked about what he wanted to accomplish. In short, he was unsatisfied about his appearance, and wanted to make changes the safest and fastest way possible. At this point, Arman was 15 years old, weighed 217lbs, had a 38-inch waist, and was 5ft 9in tall.

Arman finally had the goals he needed to focus on, and I started working with him throughout his dramatic weight loss. We developed an effective exercise routine that worked for his schedule, and what he wanted to accomplish. Obviously, he needed a plan that focused on weight loss and tone. With that in mind, we designed effective cardio and weight lifting sessions to get the job done. After 4 months of hard work and body sculpting, Arman lost 4 inches in his waist. Arman and I did not focus too much on weight when we started; however, during February of 2009, we discovered he lost 37lbs. His confidence began to grow, as did his knowledge of what it would take to reach his goals.

After learning of his capabilities, Arman decided to re-evaluate his goals, and defined what he wanted even more. In August 2009, he lost another 2 inches, and was able to get into a size 32. We did not know what his exact target was, so we based results on weight loss, inches lost, and muscle tone. We were making our way into uncharted territory. Arman had never had a specific workout plan for his body, and we were discovering what was possible for his physique. We focused a bit more on the weights, cardio, and diet in specific areas. In June of 2009, Arman lost a total of 52lbs and maintained a consistent weight of 165lbs.

It is important to understand weight loss from different angles. If a person starts going to the gym, and then loses weight, he/she has conquered a great feat. However, the real question is, can that person keep the weight off? What is the point of losing weight, if you do not plan to keep it off? You should only have to do it once, right? Arman changed his LIFESTYLE to lose his excess weight, and did not focus only on his weight loss. Without a doubt, losing weight can be a great accomplishment. Unfortunately, if you do not plan to change your lifestyle and commit to keep the weight off, all of your efforts will be in vain. If I had to lose the same weight over and over again, I would not be motivated to keep going through the constant disappointment either. In other words, if you are out of shape, it is because of the lifestyle you are living. You need to live healthy to be healthy. Live a healthy lifestyle, and stop complicating your situation. Try living a healthy lifestyle, and watch what happens to your body after a few months.

Arman learned a very important lesson during his transition. When a person wants to get results, it takes time, consistency, the willingness to change, and dedication. He learned that you must test yourself to learn of your capabilities. He learned that you must pursue something fully to say that, at the very least, you have tried, and at the most, succeeded. He learned that his health is equally important as his education. Arman also learned how the environment of a person has a tremendous impact of the decisions they make. The most important thing he learned was that he is capable of achieving great triumphs by committing to his goals.

As I watched Arman overcome his struggle with his weight, I learned that an individual couldn't make the best of any journey without direction and support. Through his experience, I have learned what true success means. True success comes from applying yourself to accomplish what you want to do in life. If you want to be successful in life, you have to show up to the starting line first. There are many people who want to lose weight and get in shape, but they never get off the couch. I applaud Arman for showing up to the starting line, and ultimately finishing with his success.

Testimonial from Arman Moeini:

If you are reading this, you are more or less in a position where you are considering taking a life-changing course to better yourself. That course is laced with hard work, sweat, pain, self-control, and many emotions that will not agree with your body. But I promise you, if you undertake this journey, you will not regret any bit of your fight. Beyond looking and feeling healthy, younger, more vibrant, the path to your ultimate goal absolutely consumes you into self-discovery that you cannot ignore. You will learn your limits, you will impress yourself, you will see what patience, and yes I mean extreme patience, and hard work and hope can do for you. You will have the confidence and know-how to undertake any other goal in life, and carefully plan short-term, intermediate, and long-term goals to make the most of this one chance you have. Honestly, you can only go up from here. So take the risk. Prove not only to yourself, but everyone, that you can accomplish anything you set your mind to. Most importantly, chart your success with photos and logs. When it is all said and done, there is nothing more satisfying than looking back where you came from and where you stand at the finish line.

-Arman Moeini

There are many ways to approach an exercise routine. When it comes to personal fitness, it would be wise for you to focus on what will work best for your lifestyle. Think about it, does your lifestyle stay the same all the time? No, it does not. The wrong exercise routine may cost valuable time, and bring you frustration when you are not making desired progress. Going to your place of fitness, with an actual plan, is a big step in terms of progress.

Exercising in vain can cause boredom, and erode your commitment level. Hire a Personal Trainer when you have educated yourself as much as possible, and can no longer tolerate the monotonous field trips to the gym. Some people need personal trainers and some people do not. Some people like to have exercise partners. Some people like to go solo. Everyone needs something different. There are many ways to achieve your goal, and everyone will not use the same approach. Become a student of what you want to master, by putting in the time and effort to learn it. Avoid trying multiple approaches at once, and take note of the ones that interest you the most. By having options, you will have greater interest in what you are doing. By having greater interest, you will have the ability to achieve better results. You will not put your all into something in which you do not have an intense interest.

Education

How do you educate yourself about fitness? Education can be attained from the many sources you have in your every day life. In regards to fitness education, knowing the subject of your education is most important. You will gather the subject of your education from your goals. What did you put down for your goals? If you wrote down weight loss for a goal, research different weight loss techniques. If you wrote down weight gain, research different weight gain techniques. There are many reliable information sources available for your fitness interest, if you take the time to look. Sources of fitness education include the Internet, books, exercise videos, exercise television, magazines, and a qualified health or fitness professional.

As I mentioned earlier, fitness education will give you the tools to accomplish your personal goals with consistency and purpose. Focus on the details of your goals to identify the techniques you need to learn. Gather the techniques that interest you, and compare them to the goals you want to accomplish. There should be a connection between the techniques and your goals. If your goal is to run faster, the techniques you should study are the ones describing how to increase your speed. You can explore your options by educating yourself. By exploring your options, you find the best techniques that work for your goals and your lifestyle. Write down the techniques (with brief descriptions) you will practice in the blank lines on the next page. When your goals change, you will need to research new techniques.

Exercise Techniques

Consulting Your Doctor

"Consult your doctor before you begin any exercise routine, conditioning, or stretching routine". We see this statement frequently; yet, we overlook its importance. The National Institute of Health advises all persons to consult their doctor, and a health care professional before beginning any exercise program, to avoid exercising improperly. Consulting with a doctor before engaging in physical activity is something most people ignore, because we all think we are "ok". Consequently, if you have not exercised in a very long time, your body may not be able to handle certain types of stress in its present condition. When you consult your doctor about exercising, he/she will be able to tell you what you can and should not do in your current state of health. It is very easy to over-exert when you are not aware of your true physical condition. If your body is accustomed to walking and limited functional motions, it is not prepared to exert energy out of normal parameters. Let me give you an example. Most cars can accelerate to speeds up to 120 miles per hour. However, we rarely drive them at their top speed. When we try to drive faster, we notice there is an uneasy sense of having control. If we continue driving at a speed we cannot handle, we will crash eventually. Be smart about beginning your exercise routine. Consult your doctor

or physician for clearance to exercise. Ensuring your vehicle is ready to drive will help you avoid a crash. To eliminate injuries, you must first condition your body to handle certain types of stress.

Physical Conditioning and Overtraining

Conditioning your body before engaging in a regular physical routine or intense event is very important. Over time, our body becomes accustomed to the movements we perform daily. If you make an attempt to step out of that zone, your body does not hesitate to let you know that it is not ready for the transition. Transitioning from one fitness level to the next is where physical conditioning has its purpose. Your body will not perform a task to which it is not accustomed, without risk of injury. Can you think of a time when your muscles were so sore, that it hurt to walk or laugh? If you ignore prevention, you can tear muscles, ligaments, and inflict other types of bodily damage without proper conditioning. Injury prevention is one of the reasons why warming up, stretching, and conditioning are all very important aspects of fitness. From personal experience, I find that a light warm up before stretching allows the body to make a smooth transition into exercising.

How do I condition my body? You can start by increasing your general fitness. If you increase your endurance, strength, and flexibility before your specific conditioning, you can transition effectively into the conditioning for your specific techniques of interest. After you increase your general fitness, then take some time to study the techniques that have your interest. What do those techniques require: strength, endurance, and flexibility? The way you condition your body will be more effective, if you couple it with the activities you will soon engage with your body. By preparing your muscles for your future actions, your muscles will be accustomed to the function, and allow you to make a smooth transition to the next phase of your exercise routine.

Conditioning should last as long as it takes. Unless you have an event coming up, there is no need to rush your body into intense performance. The body can perform any task better, if it is allowed to make a smooth transition into that task. When you think of any professional sports team, the players always go through a period of conditioning after the off-season. During the off-season, it is rare to find an athlete that maintains his/her playing level. In any case, it is good to give the body a rest after a long period of intense physical activity. Conditioning will not alleviate all the aches and pains that may accompany physical activity, but is a vital tool for injury protection.

Overtraining can happen to anyone. Naturally, when we get results, sometimes we think more is better. On the contrary, our muscles need rest between workouts. Having pain or soreness, is not necessarily a good thing. Although it is normal to experience soreness after a hard workout, you should consult your doctor if it lingers. You can reach your goals without overtraining your body and risking damage. Mix up your routine by having intense days and moderate days. Study your techniques and routines to pursue the right type of conditioning and avoid overtraining. You will be glad you did. Leave the intense conditioning, and training for the people who need it to do their jobs. If you are not lifting 400lbs every day at your job, then why is it so important for you lift that weight? It may be a great accomplishment, but is it worth the injury? Think smart about preserving your body, and ensure that the benefits always outweigh the risks.

Fitness Centers

To many of us, the gym is a place of conditioning, fitness, and the means to accomplishing our exercise goals. Going to a gym is a very simple process, but using the gym efficiently is very complex.

Most of us are not aware of the nature of a gym. We sign a contract for a year or more, and say to ourselves that we use the facility as many times as possible. From my experience as a Personal Trainer, I can tell you that most individuals do not have goals as they walk into the gym; yet, individuals continue to perform specific exercises with the hope of making great progress. Physical accomplishments are limited in the gym without self-education and a concrete plan.

There are some individuals who become very intimidated and confused when they enter a gym. Believe me, I understand what you feel. When you walk into a gym, there are so many people doing various routines on so many different machines. Where do you start? How do you start? What area do you stay in or avoid? I will tell you where you start. You start with the techniques you learned. Start your journey to health and fitness with something you already know. Familiarity is a great way to develop confidence and focus. Would it surprise you that the majority of the members of the gym have little understanding of the routines they practice? With that being said, there is no need to be confused or intimidated. You have done your research and educated yourself; you know exactly what to do. Do not worry about those fancy machines, and what everyone else is doing.

What someone else is trying to accomplish is irrelevant to your personal goals. Practice what you know, and learn more about other techniques as you become more interested. Repeat the process to expand your knowledge of fitness.

After getting approval from your doctor, and after conditioning your body, you will be able to perform your techniques of interest in a gym setting or at home. With proper study and practice of the techniques you researched, you will then be able to attain your desired results. At this point, your next plan of action should involve utilizing a health professional.

Personal Trainers

If you are taking this journey seriously, I suggest that you consider hiring an experienced Personal Trainer, to learn effective exercise routines. Personal Trainers assist you in accomplishing exercise goals you would otherwise not accomplish on your own. Trainers assist you in surpassing your limits safely, and teach you new concepts of fitness that really work; notice I keep saying "assist". A trainer cannot watch over you without being in your presence; therefore, he/she has a limited role. Learning effective exercises and effective routines from a qualified professional will cut down on time wasted, and keep you moving in the right direction towards your goals. Think of hiring a trainer as an investment in your personal health education. Over many years, you have invested thousands of dollars into your college education, cars, trips, and your home. You should be more than willing to invest money in your health, the return on this investment is greater than you can imagine, and you collect tremendously on the back end. Closely related, being educated in the area of fitness is just like having a college education. You have a much greater possibility to accomplish more when you have it.

When choosing a Personal Trainer, you want to seek a trainer that compliments your personality, understands your goals, and one who can motivate you. It is a personal relationship, and you want to have a good relationship with someone who is educating you. After all, you should plan to be with him/her for at least one month. There are a few topics to consider when you want to hire a Personal Trainer.

1. Experience
2. Education
3. Training Philosophy
4. Conduct and Appearance
5. Personality and Motivation

6. Clientele

7. Location

8. Schedule

9. Pricing

10. Parting Ways with Your Trainer

Experience – Experience is the most important attribute you should seek in a Personal Trainer. When you think about it, it is a great feeling to know that your best interests are being considered. With that being said, an experienced Personal Trainer will get to know you on a personal level, and will assess you by doing a thorough evaluation. After all, how can a trainer start you on a program without knowing whom you are, where you want to go, and the status of your current fitness level? In any case, a trainer should be able to put you on the right plan after meeting with you two to three times. Unfortunately, it is impossible for your trainer to assist you in accomplishing much at all, if you are unable to establish and then share your goals with him or her. On that note, you should determine your goals, not your Personal Trainer. A trainer does not have much to work with when you say "I just want to get in shape". When you give your trainer a broad goal, you do not give him/her a specific target. Remember, your trainer works for you and with you. You tell them what you want, and then they tell you if they can deliver, or if it is possible at all.

There is also another side of the trainer to client relationship. If you do not have the motivation, or you know you will not exercise on your own, a Personal Trainer is a great option. Your Personal Trainer will guide you through a great workout each time you meet with him/her. Knowing what you need from a Personal Trainer is critical, and not knowing what you need from a Personal Trainer can make your relationship with them indefinite. Ask yourself the following question: Do you need your trainer to assist you in maintaining your current fitness level or help you get to a certain goal? Know what you need before you meet with a Personal Trainer. I have trained some individuals for several years, and some for only a few weeks. When you think of having a Personal Trainer in your life, would you want your trainer to be a consistent fitness motivator, or get you to a certain goal you wish to attain?

There is a big difference in having a fitness motivator and someone training you for a specific goal. When you use your trainer as a fitness motivator, you may not have the motivation to make time for your exercise routine, and you want to incorporate their expertise into your lifestyle. You may also want a trainer as a fitness motivator because they help you train in the areas you have trouble with. When you use your trainer to assist you in achieving your goals, he/she becomes a catalyst for you, by adding an extra spark to everything you are working hard for. Using a trainer as a fitness motivator or catalyst can last as little as one month or many years. Either is a good option, if you know what you want.

Education – The education of the trainer you choose is very important, and the trainer you choose should be certified in what you want to focus on. A Personal Trainer certification is a requirement for him/her to train you in a physical manner. However, this education needs to be coupled with experience. A trainer needs education from the book and from people they have trained. When it all boils down, it is you who knows what you want, and the trainer knows what you need. If you believe you want to have core training only, you should train with a certified personal trainer who is certified in core training and/or has the experience. In some cases, you may have a trainer who is certified in a specific area, who also trains the area in which you want to improve. For example, if you have someone who is a boxing fitness instructor, he/she also teaches core training. Boxing strengthens the core tremendously. When you are looking for a trainer with a certain expertise, just ask them about their certifications. If they do not have a certain certification, ask them about their experience. It is your job to make an informed decision about hiring a personal trainer.

Training Philosophy- All trainers have a different training philosophy, which is based upon their knowledge, experience, and understanding of how to be an effective Personal Trainer. When you hire a trainer, and then work with a different trainer later, you will notice their philosophies are quite different. The current trainer you hired will give you advice that contradicts what you learned from your previous trainer. Think about it. Of course the two trainers will give different advice, as they have had different education and experience. Neither is wrong and it is up to you to realize that each trainer has a different style. If you are thinking about what your past trainer taught you, your current trainer will not be able to make any progress with you. Excluding bodily harm, there is no such thing as a wrong way to train; only a more effective way to achieve a specific goal. Depending on your goal, there may be a more efficient or effective way, which is why it is important to interview your trainer so that you may understand their style of training.

Conduct and Appearance - Appearance is important when you know what to look for. Appearance should be taken into account when it comes to professionalism. Obviously, professionalism is important in any profession. I am sure you would not feel confident hiring a personal trainer that could not utilize the same discipline they are teaching you.

A personal trainer does not need to be extremely buff or cut to exhibit their understanding of fitness. However, they should practice what they preach. A trainer will not understand the full magnitude of a given training style, unless he/she has experienced that style of training personally. On the other hand, you could have a trainer with an incredible physique, but lacking knowledge to aid you in achieving your goals. A qualified trainer does not necessarily have to look like a Greek statue. On the other hand, he/she should not appear or act uncaring about the health of their body. However, if you feel he/she does not look the part, it is a possibility they could have a valid reason. Maybe they are in the process of losing weight themselves, and are trying to teach others how they have done it. That trainer could have lost 200lbs, but to you they may seem unqualified. In fact, they are qualified, they have personal experience, and they may know how you feel. The old saying "Don't judge a book by its cover" has meaning. When choosing a trainer, get to know them so you may learn about their struggles and motivations; INTERVIEW.

Personality and Motivation– We all respond differently to certain types of personalities. You may not like it if someone yelled at you, told you what to do, or told you to stop being lazy. You also may not like it if someone treated you like a baby, did not push you, or stopped when they thought things were getting too tough for you. Do you need someone to push you harder when you do not have any strength left? Do you need someone to have patience? When you find out what you need, you will be able to match it with the right type of trainer personality. When it is right, it will feel right. The right trainer will discover what pushes you and motivates you, by getting to know you. An experienced Personal Trainer has a keen sense of observing, and will adjust when the situation requires it.

When you think of hiring a Personal Trainer, you want to know that the person cares about your goals. A caring Personal Trainer invests a tremendous amount of time in you. Your trainer should be eager to learn more about who you are as a person, what your obstacles are, and what you really need and want from your exercise routine. Obviously, if a trainer leaves you hanging without direction, you probably will not go very far with them. I have met many Personal Trainers in the past, and I have found more dedication in the trainer with an emotional attachment to their profession. I am not discrediting other fitness professionals in any way. I am pointing out the significance of the relationship you may need to establish with a trainer who is helping you reach your goal. If you lost a good friend because of the unhealthy lifestyle they lived, then you probably will connect more with a trainer who has lost a friend or family member in the same way. When you need that type of personal trainer, you should seek them, and not someone looking at you as another client for the books. How do you identify a trainer with this type of dedication? Interview your personal trainer, and listen to their story. They could have had a personal experience, family experience, or an experience that sparked something inside of them. When you hire a Personal Trainer who chose the profession because they are good at their job that may not be enough to get you to your goal.

Clientele – If you are referred to a trainer by a friend, and you are impressed with their accomplishments, you should have a good idea of the capabilities of that Personal Trainer. If you set up a meeting with a trainer, ask them to show you pictures of their clients who gave that trainer permission to show their progress. Listen to the trainer describe how the client achieved those results, and identify with a situation that sounds like yours. If you do not like what you see or hear, interview another trainer. You can avoid disappointment by paying attention to signs of incompatibility. Follow your intuition when you meet your trainer.

Location – Contrary to what most people believe, you do not need a gym to exercise. On the television, we see fitness commercials filmed in the gym most of the time. From personal experience, I have learned that most of the better workouts take place outside of the gym, or in an environment where you must manipulate your body in an unconventional manner. An experienced personal trainer can train you at home, and without most weights. If you are short on time, find a place close to you, or find a trainer who can come to your home. If you are flexible on time, find a place that is close to a park. This way, when you get tired of the gym, you can take your workouts outside.

Schedule – Most trainers maintain the time of their sessions between thirty and sixty minutes. Thirty minutes is plenty of time for you to get a great workout. According to the Center of Disease Control, on a weekly basis, adults need 2 hours and 30 minutes of moderate aerobic activity, and 2 days or more of muscle strengthening exercises. The Center of Disease Control also points out that you can participate in 1 hour and 15 minutes of vigorous aerobic activity accompanied by 2 or more days of muscle strengthening exercises, and receive the benefits for body as well.

If you have not had an intense workout in some time, only do a 30-minute session; do not pay for 1 hour when you can only last 35 minutes. On the same lines, I would advise you to refrain from scheduling your time with a Personal Trainer around your busiest time of the day. When you are training, you need to be there physically and mentally. You will not stay focused if you have somewhere else to be. Do not pay for the education if you are not going to attend the class.

Pricing – When you think of how much you should pay for a personal training session, think of how much money you have spent on things in your lifetime previously. How much did you pay for your car? How much did you pay for your education? How much did you pay for your wedding? The list goes on and on. When you take a look at all of these things you have purchased, do any of them have a direct impact on your health in a positive way? Most of us will say "no". Why have you not invested money into something that will allow you to live longer? Well, I hate to break the news to you. You have to be healthy if you want to utilize, and enjoy all of the great things in your life. Without your health, materialistic and educational gains mean absolutely nothing. Invest in what it takes to maintain your health. How much is your health worth to you? You are the judge in this situation.

On the low scale, you can expect to pay one dollar per minute with a personal trainer. On a high scale you can expect to pay almost twice as much. It depends on where you are, and who your trainer is. Think of this decision in a logical way. You can pay the person who charges you a low rate, and hire them for up to six months to get what you need. Or you can pay on the high end, hire the person for one month, and get the same results. In all actuality, it evens out. How much money you pay is hardly a factor. Furthermore, if you do not have a goal, you cannot invest wisely in your fitness education.

Parting Ways with Your Trainer- As you work with your trainer for some time, you will notice a relationship of trust and honesty develops. Naturally, problems arise with every relationship. As we all know, effective communication is key. If you have a problem with your trainer let them know immediately. He/she cannot read your mind. Unfortunately, at some point, you will feel it is time for you to part ways with your trainer. Here are a few common reasons why people part ways with their trainer.

1. You reached your goal
2. Lost interest
3. Trainer is not effective anymore
4. Change in financial situation
5. Need a different training style

You may also need to be aware of the commitment on your end. If your trainer writes a plan for you, and you ignore it, there is not much he/she can do with your progress. If you do not follow your plan for reaching your goals, which includes training on our own, you are not going to make much progress. In a relationship with a Personal Trainer, most of the effort comes from your end, and you must understand your responsibility. I commend any Personal Trainer who can achieve significant physical changes, without the person doing any work on their own; this trainer has a very effective program. Unfortunately, not giving 100% also means you are only getting a portion of the results you could get.

Previously, I mentioned that if you are not ready to commit to a Personal Trainer, do not hire one. After all, if you are to gain any success from a Personal Trainer, commitment must be present. For the sake of success, commitment involves your listening intently to their instructions, accepting their training style, maintaining a healthy diet, and exercising more on your own than with your trainer. The only exception is if you are using your trainer as a fitness motivator; at this point, you have accepted that you will not exercise much when you are alone. Alternatively, doing a little exercise is better than doing none at all.

Unfortunately, it is necessary to part ways in some cases. In any event, if the bridge is not intact on both ends you cannot make it to your destination. If this is the case, do not waste your time or your trainer's time.

Exercise: Questions for a Personal Trainer

There are many questions you should ask a Personal Trainer. The questions you ask a trainer should help you learn more about him/her, if they can help you reach your goals, and if they are a good match for you.

1. Why did you choose to become a Personal Trainer?

_____

_____

_____

2. How long have you been a Personal Trainer?

_____

_____

3. What is your training philosophy?

_____

_____

_____

4. How long will it take me to reach my goals?

_____

_____

_____

5. Will I have to go on a diet? Why?

_____

_____

_____

_____

6. What is the most important thing to consider when starting an

exercise program?

_____

_____

7. What should I expect to feel and experience during our first

month together?

_____

_____

_____

8. How much are your sessions?

_____

_____

_____

_____

9. How many times will we train during one week? Why?

_____

_____

_____

_____

10. May I see some of your training accomplishments?

11. What are your current certifications?

_____

_____

_____

_____

_____

12. What separates you from other Personal Trainers?

_____

_____

_____

_____

_____

These simple questions will help you develop a good foundation with your trainer. To gather more info, you may ask as many as you want. After all, you want to make sure you are making the right investment. As I mentioned previously, these questions are to help you understand, and get to know your trainer better. After you know more about him/her, you will be in a position to make an informed decision about hiring them or not.

Utilizing a Personal Trainer

After you have decided on the trainer that suits you best, you can then move on to the next step of going through an evaluation with your trainer. In this stage, the trainer should establish your current physical condition through a series of tests. As I mentioned earlier, a trainer cannot assist you in reaching your goal, if they do not know the status of your fitness level. We all feel strong and tough, until we are put to the test. After your evaluation, you will know your true strength and endurance. To clarify, your evaluation should consist of strength, stabilization, core, flexibility, and endurance exercises. The tests will let you know your limits in certain areas. Think of it as riding a bike. You do not know how to adjust and balance the bike, until you get on it. In the same way, you will not know how to exercise properly until you start a routine and get the feel for it. With an effective assessment, your trainer will help you reach your limits safely, without putting too much stress on your body.

I do not recommend utilizing your trainer every day, unless you are preparing for a special event that requires intense training, or you are using them as a fitness motivator. Unfortunately, the drawback on utilizing a trainer daily is developing a dependency. If that is not the case, in my opinion, three days a week is the max. If you are truly seeking success, you should get use to exercising on your own. You should be able to push yourself most of the time. The job of your trainer is to keep you motivated and focused on the goals you are trying to accomplish. Your trainer is not responsible for your progress, or the achievement of your goals. In terms of responsibility, you have to take ownership of your goals, and put in the extra work when you are not with your trainer.

I will give you examples of how to develop an effective schedule with your trainer. These examples are not to be used as a routine. Your exercise routine should come from a qualified Personal Trainer whom you have interviewed. Use the example only to clarify and understand how to develop a consistent exercise routine with your trainer.

Let's pretend you are on a consistent schedule with your trainer.

Monday- Trainer

Tuesday- Personal workout routine from trainer

Wednesday- Trainer

Thursday – Personal workout routine from trainer

Friday – Personal workout routine from trainer

When your trainer gives you instructions, he/she must know what equipment you are able to use for your solo workouts, and how much time you are willing to commit to exercise. You need to develop an exercise routine that compliments your lifestyle. If you only have 30mins for working out, be sure you do not have a routine that takes an hour.

When you start an individual exercise routine, it should compliment what you are doing with your Personal Trainer. Along the same lines, your trainer should instruct and teach you about proper form, and reasons for doing certain exercises. In the end, when you are performing your exercises solo, you should be totally confident in what you are doing, because you have learned the right techniques from your trainer. You should be confident about having the right form, and that you are doing what will work best for you.

Once you have the correct exercise routines, you can exercise anywhere. You may not need to become a member of a gym to exercise. You will have the ability to exercise in your garage, in your living room, at the park, on the beach, and any of the other locations you choose to. The local gym is a great place, but offers you limited tools to use your body in a functional manner. Keep in mind, you have unlimited options for exercising when you have the knowledge. Use your knowledge, and do not worry about having a gym membership to get the job done. I would recommend learning the skills to exercise without a gym, before you get a gym membership. With this type of awareness you will not limit yourself to the gym environment, and you will not make excuses to skip your workouts. Your progress is limited only by what you know and what you have not learned.

Once you have a good grasp of your routine, you have unlimited potential. You will be able to go into the gym, and know what you have to do to get your desired results. Think of it this way, when you have a trainer, you get educated. When you get educated, you make better decisions, and get better results. Once you learn what you need from your trainer, continue your routine on your own. When you need help again, call your trainer to get you back on track. Let me give you an example. You maintain your hair as much as you can on a daily basis, right? When you cannot maintain your hair anymore, you go to a stylist or a barber. Utilizing a Personal Trainer is not any different. After all, most of us cannot afford Personal Trainers for an extended period. If you are going to utilize a trainer, get the most out of your experience: attention, education, and motivation. A Personal Trainer cannot provide you with much more. Most of the hard work, commitment, and dedication must come from you.

Notes

_____

_____

_____

_____

_____

_____

_____

_____

_____

_____

_____

_____

Step 5

Proper Nutrition

When you think of eating healthy, what images come to your mind? For many individuals, a healthy meal is a boring plate of tasteless food, void of exciting flavors. For some people, healthy food takes too much time to prepare, because we prefer to eat quickly. In contrast, for those health conscious minds, healthy foods are the way to really enjoy your meals, and get those special flavors that only come from nutritious foods.

As we gather a sense of what foods we like, over time, most people customize their meals with certain foods they desire. It is perfectly normal to want food with flavor, variety, and different texture. Naturally, we all want to eat food that excites our taste buds. Due to our fast paced world, fast food chains can manipulate an individual by having fast foods that are bursting with artificial flavors. The quick meals do not stop there, and they are available in the grocery store in almost every aisle. There is not much nutritional value we can gather from highly processed foods. If you think about it, the nutritional value is what is most important when selecting your foods. Sadly, the average person spends little time understanding what nutritious foods can do for their bodies, and more time on how it can make them feel emotionally. In fact, the average person does not look at the nutrition label at all. When it boils down to us being at the grocery store, we think about buying something that satisfies us with that specific flavor we are looking for, especially, when we are eating alone.

In traditional settings, eating is a social event and the dining room is a gathering point for friends and family. For some of us, food is a comfort tool, used to calm us down during those stressful times. When we are on the go, eating is an event we want to spend little time doing, because we are just too busy. Sadly, there are a few of us who would prefer not to eat, out of fear of gaining weight. Let us approach these four topics on a "common sense" level. The goal of this chapter is to provide you with insight on the different types of eating habits, not to provide solutions for personal issues with food consumption. Please consult a dietician for expert advice.

1. Social Eating

Imagine going out to your favorite restaurant, it is rare that you see someone eating their meal in solitude. In fact, eating has mostly been a social event throughout history, as we all know from our personal experiences. When we have parties, there seems to be an unlimited amount of food, ready for the taking. Whenever we celebrate a major accomplishment, there is always food for the occasion. For any special occasion, food remains the constant.

Eating out, or eating at special events provides an individual with a unique environment. The individual is placed in an environment, in which they can eat as much as they can stuff in their bodies (literally). The food is tasteful, but also full of extra calories. When we place ourselves in these environments, our awareness of overeating tends to go down. On the other hand, why should we focus on our eating habits during this time? We are having fun, and spending time with people we like being around. I totally agree, when you are having fun with friends, family, or dating, you should eat the foods you want at that time.

The act of "eating out" is not a major issue. The real issue is eating out multiple times during the same day and week. Ponder with me for a moment, if you will. If you exercised, and ate nutritious foods most of the week, why would one day be an issue? You can eat at your favorite restaurant, but not every day. Eating out everyday, and binge eating, are consistencies that get the best of us. We seem to do it unconsciously, and with total disregard. Unfortunately, over time, the extra calories add up, and so do the pounds. Did you know that 3500 calories equals one pound of fat? If you eat out multiple times during the week and go to enough parties, you will surely pick up those extra pounds easily. During one month you could gain up to 5 or 10lbs. For the majority of us, gaining 5 to 10lbs in a month, usually happens over the holiday season. When the holiday season arrives, have you noticed how your weight starts going up, and it does not want to come down? During the holiday season, we are eating unconsciously in a social setting, and attending various holiday parties. What can you do?

The best equation for avoiding excess calories is limiting your binge eating and eating out. To those of us who rarely eat out or go to parties, the subject of eating out too much may not be an issue. For the rest of us, calorie consumption and consideration is necessary. How many extra calories will you eat this week?

2. Comfort Food

Comfort Food is exactly what it sounds like. Comfort food seems to take stress out of the day, and allows us to relax. Every individual has a comfort food, which seems to float around in our minds, when we have certain feelings. Have you ever been in a situation, in which you were cold, and you wanted something warm to eat; like soup? Have you ever walked on the beach, during the summer, and suddenly wanted ice cream? We like comfort foods, because we can get them easily, and they satisfy the way we are feeling at the current moment. In most cases, you will find that a comfort food is something you can grab and eat quickly with easy access. A certain food could not comfort us if we had to wait on it, right?

The problem with indulging in a comfort food is the possibility of eating until you are totally satisfied with that one food. Imagine being hungry, and your comfort food is chocolate chip cookies. You could eat an entire bag of chocolate chip cookies, because you are hungry, and indulging in a comfort food. I will let you do the calculation of the calorie consumption for that scenario. If you eat your normal meal before you eat comfort foods, you will most likely not over-indulge in that type of food.

There is a simple way to control comfort foods. Find your favorite comfort foods, and put a visual on them. After you discover them, ask yourself, what is it about that specific food item that comforts you? Find a healthier alternative that can give you the same comfort. You can find alternatives by experimenting with different foods. It will take some time to find healthy foods that will comfort you, but you can do it with discipline. In my opinion, there is nothing wrong with having a comfort food, if it is healthy for you. Did you know that you could avoid unhealthy foods if you did not buy them? Have you ever thought about not buying those bad foods? After all, if they are not in the house you cannot eat them. Please do not use the kids as an excuse.

3. Don't Have Time

There are many reasons why a person may not take time to eat. Unfortunately, those reasons do not qualify as valid excuses. Most people know it is a necessity to fuel your body with proper nutrition, right? Wrong! There are some people that simply forget to eat. Examine the list below. Could this have been you this week?

1.   The person with a closing deadline on a big project
2.   The student with major exams approaching

3.   The person worried about a sick family member

4.   The person starting a new job tomorrow

5.   The child that starts his/her first day of school

At times in our lives, it is natural to get so busy or distracted that we forget to put nutrients I our body's. However, it is not natural for you to keep letting it happen. If you feel that your schedule will not allow you to eat, something must change. Put yourself on an eating schedule. If you can commit to deadlines and schedules, so why not put yourself on an eating schedule with deadlines? Skipping a meal is not an option. Your body needs nutrients to function properly. Sure, I know your job is important, or you do not feel like eating, but your body needs the necessary nutrients to function; it is not an open discussion. From where will the nutrients come if you do not eat? Will they formulate in your body at your wishing? They certainly will not. Each of us has specific duties to perform in our daily lives. How is it possible that you can perform at your highest potential, without your body performing at its highest potential? Does it make sense to skip meals, and then load your body with energy supplements to get the boost you need? SIT DOWN AND EAT A MEAL! The body is a fine piece of work and can remain that way if you respect it. I know, without deadlines, nothing would finish on time. Think of the deadlines your body has. Think of everything that must happen for you to take one step with your foot. Respecting your body is one deadline you do not want to miss.

4. I Do Not Like To Eat

I have met people who have admitted that they prefer not to eat. They feel that one full meal will cause them to gain a significant amount of weight. If you believe you might fit into this category, you could convince yourself that minimal consumption of food is a healthy option. However, I would ask you to consider learning about bodily functions, and why nutrients are so important in this process.

Media and fashion have forced us to believe that a certain look is beautiful. Did you know that most of the images on the cover of magazines are computer enhanced? That fact means that the person on that cover does not exist! When do you think the fashion world will design clothes that actually fit the normal person? Yes, you guessed right, they will not. Have you noticed that all the models have the same body type?

If you are not eating because you are not happy with the way you look, welcome to the club! Guess what, no one is completely happy with the way they look. We all deal with this constant disappointment daily, and choose to do different things about it; exercise, dieting, and cosmetic surgery. Nevertheless, the smarter decision would be to do something that is conducive to our health, and actually adds value to us. Making a decision to starve your body does not fall into a healthy category. I hope it is a clear understanding that starving your body is not in any way beauty enhancing; nor is it conducive in sustaining a healthy life.

Nutritious Foods

For a basic understanding what foods to eat, you will need to understand the value of vitamins and minerals. Conduct your own research and develop a list of vitamins, minerals, and a listing of foods containing them. As you develop this list of vitamins, minerals, and food choices, you can easily develop your personal combination of healthy foods that satisfy your taste buds. While doing your research, you will not find microwaveable meals or meal replacements; only the individual food choices. From a young age most children are taught the value of nutrient dense foods. Unfortunately, as we become busier, we seek convenience. Naturally, we find ourselves eating the same foods every day that lack nutrient density for the sake of saving time. It sounds like common sense, but you can overlook nutrition if you continue to buy "convenience" foods. You have a better chance of getting the nutrients you need by varying your choices with natural foods.

Most of us know that nutritious food comes from the earth, and does not grow in plastic bags, or microwaveable dishes. Yet, because we are always in a rush and looking for something with guaranteed flavor, we take the lesser option. I want you to do a quick exercise. Go to your pantry and select any food item from the shelf. Go ahead! Get it now! Look on the back, where the "Nutrition Facts" are. Can you identify the listed ingredients? If someone showed you what those ingredients were individually, could you recognize them? Can you pronounce the words? If you do not know what it is, chances are your body does not recognize it either. You will notice these strange ingredients on most of your highly processed foods. Fortunately, not all processed foods are bad; however, if you are going to put something in your body, ensure it is something your body can use. There is a good reason why the raw vegetables do not need label, because what you see is what you get. If you see an apple, it is an apple. Eat real food; it is that simple.

If a food is considered healthy, it does not mean it will be void flavor. If you do not like vegetables or whole grains, there is a possibility that when you first encountered that particular food, you did not like the way it was prepared. Do you have a food that you enjoy when it is prepared a certain way? Yes, we all do. On the other hand, when it is prepared in other ways, we do not like it as much. Cooking vegetables requires the same attention. Experiment in your kitchen to find a vegetable recipe you like, and then add it to your list of favorite foods. Naturally, when you like the flavor of something, you tend to eat it again. If you want vegetables that actually taste good, learn how to prepare them! Get a cookbook and start experimenting. In a cookbook, you are bound to find a recipe with flavor and excitement. If you cannot get into the cookbook, go to a nice restaurant that has the foods you are confident you can enjoy, and order vegetables with your meal. If you like the vegetables you eat at the restaurant, ask your server how they were prepared, and take the recipe home. The task is not difficult at all; however, you must experiment continuously to master the process. Make smart decisions. After all, it is your body; you can pollute it or preserve it. Learn to respect your body more, by giving it the daily nutrients it needs to function first, and then leave your wants for those nutrient deficient foods last. When you are eating nutrient rich foods as a treat, your body will reward you in more ways you can imagine.

Exercise: What is my eating style?

Take a moment to answer the following questions.

1. How many times do you eat out during the week (each individual meal counts) (1-2) (3-4) (5-6) (7-8) (more than 9 times)

2. When you eat out are you aware of the calories you are consuming? Yes   No

3. Are you often mentally distracted from eating? Yes No

4. Are you eating a nutritious and balanced diet during your weekly routine? Yes No

5. The majority of the food I eat is (choose from below)
   A. Highly Processed
   B. Moderately Processed
   C. Minimally Processed
   D. All Natural

The answers to the previous questions allow you to become aware of your current situation. This insight will give you the opportunity to incorporate better decisions into your lifestyle. In most cases, your lifestyle will offer personal challenges for you, in terms of healthy eating. It is up to you to incorporate good habits of health to combat your obstacles. A busy lifestyle is not an excuse for unhealthy eating, and neither is your environment. Your awareness of this subject just took away all of your excuses.

Experiment with different foods, and then make a list of the healthy foods you like. You will find them over time, as you continually experiment. When you find something you like, write it down in the space provided below, in a journal, or create a document on your computer. There is no rush, take your time, because finding nutritious food with flavor will require a few weeks or longer. If you feel you need expert help, do not hesitate to call a registered dietician in your area.

_____

_____

_____

_____

Notes

Step 6

Journals

At this point, you should be aware of how proper nutrition serves the body. If you are not aware of what is considered proper nutrition, I encourage you to review the nutrition resources I referred to in the previous chapter. Nutrition is the second wheel on the bicycle of health. It can be misleading to think that we can exercise intensely, and then eat unhealthy foods. As you go through this journey, you will find it hard to keep track of what is working and what is not working. I suggest you use a journal to track your progress. A food and exercise journal is a great way to monitor your consistency when you find yourself falling off the path.

Visual Reference

There are times when we feel like we have done every thing we possibly can to eat better, and exercise consistently. Unfortunately, without proof to back that up, we can convince ourselves easily that it really happened. When you break down what really matters, consistency is the common denominator in everything. Your body will reflect the physical activities you are engaging in most of the time. Did you really eat healthy today, or did you eat one healthy meal and load up on comfort foods after that? With a visual, you will be able to see what you are doing exactly, and, hopefully, put an end to the frustration. Our lifestyles vary depending on the situations in which we find ourselves. During the weekday, we may eat moderately healthy, and during the weekend we may eat terribly. We may also feel like we were in the gym yesterday. With the availability of food and a busy schedule, it is easy to forget what we have eaten and how we exercised on any given day. Start a food journal and benefit from its use. If you can see it, you can beat it. By starting a journal, you will have a visual on your enemy, and eliminate it from your lifestyle.

Accountability

Without accountability we tend to lack in our ability to produce results. At our jobs, we are accountable to our boss. When health is the topic, who keeps you accountable? You should consider using your journal as an accountability log. A food and exercise journal keeps you accountable to yourself. We are all aware of the many events happening around us, what about the things happening within our personal lives. Have you ever taken a step back to observe? You can keep yourself accountable by establishing rules or limits for yourself, and teaching yourself not to cross them. Similarly, you can practice accountability by establishing goals and following up with them, by utilizing a food and exercise journal. We have a person keeping us accountable for everything in our lives, except our health. A once a year doctor visit does not count as accountability. I am talking about daily accountability. When you are starting to keep yourself more accountable, you will notice your problem areas more. They are easy to spot when you are tracking your daily actions. Unfortunately, you will not address what you are not willing to be accountable for. When you feel like you are ready for a challenge, put a visual on those problem areas, and then allow yourself to be accountable for the bad habits you have incorporated into your life.

How to track your actions

I have worked with many individuals on the subject of food journals, I have found there is no specific way you must track your progress. You must acquire a tracking system that works for you. There are some individuals who prefer to use a composition notebook, a word document, or a real journal to track their actions. If you have a phone that allows you to keep notes or track calories, you may be able to track your progress in a specific phone application. Keep your journal with you at all times, write down everything you eat, and what you do for exercise (intensity and type of exercises). Logging will only take you a few seconds (less than one minute), and then you can move on with your day. When the weekend arrives, you can take a look at your log, and judge how well you performed during the week. The results you find in your journal may surprise you. Logging a journal entry is a simple exercise you can easily do. Moreover, it does not take much time, and will prove to be very effective in your goal to become more healthy and fit.

Logging is a simple process, write the day of the week and the date in the corner of the page, then write down every thing you are eating as you consume your meals; even if its one little piece of candy. Repeat the logging process daily. I find logging to be a very useful tool in tracking my progress. Choose a method that works best for you, and then you can start the accountability process.

Summary

There are many great events that will stem from utilizing a food and exercise journal. You will be able to define your problem areas with specific details, and you will be able to see the progress you are making. Most of all, you will be able to utilize the wonderful tool of accountability.

The word accountability consists of two very important words: account and ability. Accountability for your actions means you are putting the ability to account for your actions in your hands, or giving someone or something else that ability. By being accountable, you put yourself in a position to accomplish what you feel is insurmountable.

Notes

Step 7

Obstacles

Although we can become very excited about pursuing a new goal, it is essential to consider the possible obstacles that may come along the way. There are times when it would be better to not think of the obstacles. With that being said, your journey is not one of those times. Pursuing a goal to maintain your health will require serious commitment. Furthermore, maintaining your health is not a "one time" event. It is a lifetime event. You must prepare yourself for any and every possible obstacle that may arise. I once met a young woman who did everything right, yet, still she had some of the most challenging obstacles appear in her life. Allow me to tell you another story.

During my years of training and coaching individuals, I had not imagined that one day I would have the opportunity to train a former Olympic Athlete. In a local restaurant, I was sitting across the table from Karin Deleuran, a former Olympic Swimmer. Her demeanor exuded her inner strength and focus. Across the table, I could see the intensity in her eyes as she explained to me in great detail, that she wanted to be fit again, and why it was important to her. She explained to me that she was a consistent runner, and that she had completed 3 marathons, but now she really wanted to get fit. I knew exactly what she meant; she wanted total fitness. Karin told me she wanted to tone her body, and learn to use weight training to enhance her performance in every area.

Over the span of an hour I learned more about Karin. She explained to me that she had complications with sciatica, and some limitations. I had worked with individuals with many obstacles; a person recovering from cancer, a broken foot, and fibromyalgia. Karin was the first person I had worked with, who had sciatica. She refused anything less than her full potential, and was willing to learn new and effective exercise techniques to reach her specific goal. She had no problem battling her sciatica and her additional limitations to get there.

I trained Karin for a few months and discovered the true degree of her limitations. Nevertheless, I was surprised at how much of a student she was. At that point, I learned that Karin was truly willing to learn what it would take to reach her goals. Amazingly, she was willing to forget everything she knew to open her mind to new ideas. At times, there were exercises we could not do, and at times we had to work around the intense pain in her leg. That did not stop us and we kept pushing. Determined to reach her potential, Karin pushed onward until she could no longer tolerate being limited by her sciatica. After an unfortunate experience one night, Karin decided to have back surgery to relieve the irritating sciatica condition. I trained Karin until the day of her surgery, and that is when the beginning of her nightmare began.

I did not expect to train with Karin for a few months until she had fully recovered after her surgery. Unfortunately, little did we know, it was going to take Karin months to recover. Karin went in for a simple outpatient lower back surgery on August 11, 2009, and returned home as planned later that same evening. Karin began to run a high fever, and could not walk or sleep the following days and nights. She went back to her doctor as soon as she could. Sadly, her doctor informed her that she had acquired an infection near her spine as a result of the first surgery. Karin needed to have a second surgery, and was back in the hospital on August 23rd, only 12 days after the first surgery.

Karin was put on antibiotics, as she began a long battle with a very stubborn infection. She was in and out of the hospital for months, as the infection did its worst. As the days went by, late night trips to the ER and intense pain began to consume Karin's life. After fighting for so many months, Karin was told by her new doctor that she would need a third surgery. The surgery was performed immediately on October 21. Karin nearly lost her life, and had gone to her doctor just in time. After the third surgery, new antibiotics, and 7 months later, Karin began to recover. Unfortunately, after the 7 months, she was left in a debilitated condition; unable to walk, loss of balance, and hooked up to an IV.

I had sent Karin texts during the ordeal, but never knew the magnitude of the situation. In February 2010, I told Karin we needed to exercise. She informed me that she was not in a position to exercise. I had no idea that Karin was in a wheel chair not long ago and on antibiotics (via IV) three times a day. Nevertheless, I encouraged her enough to get her to start exercising. She let me know it was going to be a challenge. When I saw her again, I could see the damage the infection had done. Karin had limited range of motion and could not make any sudden movements.

I knew Karin wanted me to be mindful of her condition, but also knew she wanted me to challenge her like the competitor she was. After an exhausting fight, she still was not ready to throw in the towel. Karin pushed harder and more intensely with her same goal in mind. She wanted to get fit, but needed to establish a new starting point. The circumstances did not matter. Karin just wanted to win her life back. Karin refused to give up, and after we practiced a few months of focused training, she was running hard again, participating in boxing fitness, and joined my intense Beach Bootcamp.

Karin taught me many important lessons throughout her experience. The first lesson was that obstacles will remain constant in your life, but you will get through them if you have a reason to fight. The second lesson was that some obstacles will challenge you to test your integrity, some will try to bury you to see if you are willing to rise to the occasion again, and some will try to drown you to see if you will come up for air. The third lesson Karin taught me was that obstacles test you to see how bad you really want to pursue your goals, if you have the tenacity to fight for what you want, or watch in fear as your dreams slip away.

The last, and most important lesson Karin taught me was to compete for your life, your dreams, and your aspirations. You only get once chance at life. You must take that chance and run with it.

Testimonial from Karin Deleuran:

The surgeon saved my life, my beautiful daughter helped me make it through each and every day, and Linton helped me get back the quality of life I thought I had lost forever. He guided and encouraged me through the exercise program he carefully developed to suit my limitations caused by the surgeries.

After my surgeries, I was a prisoner in my own body. Five months later, I started my post-surgery workouts with Linton. I began to exercise almost every day of the week, and sometimes twice a day. Now, I can run again (no marathons yet, but maybe one day...), I started participating in Linton's Beach Boot Camp twice a week, I participated in boxing fitness three times a week, I have lost 20 pounds, I am in a size 2, and best of all I can use my body again. The days are over when I got sad after seeing a person jogging in the street. I was sad because I wished it was me. I no longer feel that way, because now it is me. My wish came true, and I feel so alive again!

As an Olympic swimmer, I was fortunate enough to be coached by experienced world-class coaches from around the world. I know exactly what it means to be coached for success. The combination of Linton's professional knowledge as a Wellness Coach, combined with his amazing ability to listen, is a one of a kind formula. Linton has a unique ability to understand, motivate, and identify with his clients; and in essence make your battle his battle. Without any doubt, Linton McClain is right up there with each of the world class coaches I have known. Honestly, I actually think he is a bit ahead. Thank you Linton! I am forever grateful!

-Karin Deleuran

As I said before, the thrill of pursuing a new goal is always a great event. We are simply excited about what we are doing, and believe we will be strong enough to break through any barriers when the time comes. By all means, maintain your excitement as much as you can. It is when you are having a tough day that you will need to dig deep and find your focus, determination, and awareness to make your way around those pesky obstacles. Obstacles are just part of life, and usually make their appearance when you are trying to succeed at something. When you think you have your routine down, something comes up and destroys it all. If everything was easy, we would not get any stronger, wiser, nor would we learn from mistakes.

Obstacles come in many forms, when they relate to exercise. Your hours for work may change, or you have changed jobs. You may have a significant other come into your life, and you happily make time for them. You may have a new member of the family, a new baby, or an elder parent moving into your home. While these examples are all events that generally are viewed as happy events, they do add stress to your normal routine. Over time, events will arise in our lives that make it necessary for us to change our normal routine. What matters the most, is how we react to them. The obstacle itself is never the real issue. What matters is how we handle it. You must find a way to conquer every obstacle if you can. As time goes on, with the knowledge you gain from every obstacle you encounter and tackle along the way, you will get stronger, and the next obstacle will not appear to pose as much of a challenge to you. Did you know that obstacles are necessary hurdles for us to conquer and to show what we have learned along the journey of life? It is like a personal test, and we need to score high on it. Think about your obstacles on a larger scale. There are billions of people in the world, right? Some of those people are chasing the same goals as you. Those who find success in life, find a way to get around their obstacles. In every part of the world, there is probably someone with an obstacle so huge that it would make you laugh at your own problems, and yet, they are finding a way to win the fight. Stop wasting time worrying about things you cannot control, and focus on the things you can control. Yes, pursuing a goal can be very challenging at times, but you would not grow and develop character if all of your fights were easy.

Exercise gives you a unique opportunity to take ownership of your health. In reality, we make time, and find a way to do the things that are priorities in our lives. When the time comes, do not accept an obstacle blocking your path to success. If you make time to eat, watch your favorite show, or watch a game, then you have time to exercise. There is always time, you only have to change your priorities. Even if you did 10-minute workouts, 3 times a day, you are still getting in thirty minutes of exercise. The bottom line is, if you want to achieve something bad enough, nothing will get in your way. Answer the questions below and maneuver around those obstacles.

Exercise: My Obstacles

Answer the questions honestly and truthfully, no one is watching.

1. What are my obstacles? Write in order of how much it impacts you?

a) _____

b) _____

c) _____

d) _____

e) _____

2. What makes each one an obstacle? Explain this to yourself. Does it make sense?

_____

_____

_____

_____

_____

_____

_____

3. Which obstacles can you control? Which can you not control?

_____

_____

_____

_____

4. Obstacles are very important. They teach you a very important skill of rearranging your lifestyle to accomplish important goals in life. If there is an obstacle you cannot seem to shake, stop trying to control it. If your hours at work change, stop trying to fight it. Exercise at an available time. Unnecessary stress is UNNECESSARY.

I have a question for you. If an event in your life forces you to change your lifestyle, why would you attempt to keep the same habits? Does that make sense? If something changes in your life, you must change with the direction of your life. If you cannot change your circumstances, you must change yourself. Yes, you must make a decision to fight for what you want in life. On the other hand, you must also decide when the battle is not worth fighting. If you are a new mother or father, initially, you may fight to keep your same exercise schedule. Unfortunately, you may find that you will have to change your schedule to fit a few days of exercise into your life. There will be times in your life when you have to make decisions like the one I just described.

If you can reschedule something, or you have to tell someone "no", then do it. Your health is your number one long-term priority. Tackle the obstacles you can control and find an alternative for the obstacles in which you do not have control. Identify your obstacles, and then do what is necessary to eliminate them or incorporate them into your life.

Read this example:
Imagine yourself taking a leisurely walk through a beautiful forest. If you take a look around, you may feel the protection of towering

trees, the melody of a flowing stream, and a host of wild life all around you. You can take the time to inhale the beauty of your surroundings. In most cases, many people would enjoy being surrounded by any form of peace and serenity. I would like you to imagine this scenario in a different form. Imagine running as fast as you can through the same forest. All of a sudden, you are avoiding those beautiful trees, ducking their branches, and hopefully you will not trip over something that will take you down. A scenario can happen in your life the same way.

Have you ever made a decision to pursue something great in your life, and out of nowhere, comes a force to destroy your ambitions? I am sure you know the feeling of disappointment. Maybe you were saving money for a family vacation, and something came up to take all your savings away. Maybe you were spending quality time with your family on a regular basis, and your job started demanding more of your family time for work. Inevitably, obstacles will always come up. If you want to avoid obstacles, stay on the couch. You will not find any obstacles on the couch. Success comes with a boatload of challenges that you cannot prepare for, and must adapt to.

Sabotaging Your Progress

When you are starting to get your routine down, you may notice yourself feeling better. Your exercise schedule is starting to fit into your lifestyle. You are breathing easier during your cardio sessions, and your muscle endurance has increased. Any progress is good progress, and it means you are on your way to achieving your goals. Most of us will feel better, before we actually see any results. A few lucky individuals will see changes in a month's time. Different bodies respond to exercise differently. If your friend has an athletic build, they will probably see physical results with little effort. Just stay focused on yourself and the body you have. Your journey is about exercising with purpose, and increasing longevity. The journey is not about getting the best looking body. What seems to get an individual side-tracked the most is thinking they are finished after working out for a few weeks or months. At this point in your journey, you should understand the importance of exercising to increase your personal longevity.

How do you know your routine is working? If you were honest and true with your goals, you will see the changes you want to see in your body and energy level over a few weeks. The result will never come out the exact way you imagined it. If you recall, your goals were based upon areas you wanted to change in your life, and accomplishments that would make you feel better. These goals were logical and realistic. When you are asking yourself "Is this working", you should take a look at your initial goals. Unfortunately, many people change their goals without re-evaluating or accomplishing their initial goals. I often see a person making a goal to lose 5-10 lbs in one month. If they lose 5 lbs in three weeks, they change that goal to losing 10-15 lbs suddenly. At the end of the month they become frustrated, without acknowledging that they actually accomplished their initial goal. Stick with your plan. If your progress is moving along faster or slower than you thought it should, re-evaluate your goals when you reach the deadline. You will not get into a good routine without committing to your goals.

Its Working

Visualize yourself losing 5lbs or gaining the muscle mass you wanted. Congratulations! Did you write down how you did it? A common mistake we all make is forgetting to mark the path we took to reach a destination, and then we imprint what does not work in our minds. Each time you take a step forward, log it in your journal, and write down the steps you took to get to that point. If you lose your focus, or if something comes up in your life to keep you from exercising, you will have your notes. When you look at your notes from your log, you will smile knowing how simple it is. You will get a great recap of what has been working for you if you write down the details to your success.

While reviewing your log, you will notice different routines may work during different situations. For example, when I am under stress, I cannot exercise on my own. I find an exercise partner to keep me motivated. It is important for you to know what works for you in any given situation. When you are keeping your food and exercise log, it is a good idea to keep track of your lifestyle during that week. Write down important notes about your behavior. Allow me to give you a sample what it means to properly log your weekly challenges.

Week 1

Obstacles:

Schedule changed at work

My son just started the soccer season

I only exercised once this week

Week 2:

Obstacles:

Schedule change and soccer season

I am going in an hour later but staying 2 hours more

Tried to workout in the morning; was able to get 3 workouts this week.

Week 3:

Obstacles:

None

I actually like working out in the mornings better.

I exercised 5 times this week and I feel great.

Write this brief weekend summary in your food and exercise log. These notes will help you keep track of what was actually happening in your life during a certain period, and show you how you conquered the obstacles. The next time an obstacle appears in your life, you can look back in the past and see how you handled it.

Complacency

When you get close to reaching your goal, it is easy to become complacent. When your workouts start to get easier and you stop sweating as much, you must bring the intensity back. Too many times I have seen an individual become disappointed, because they have reached a plateau. ***You are not supposed to keep practicing the same exercise routines***. Do you really think the same 30 minutes on the elliptical will give you different results over a 12-month period? You have to get comfortable being uncomfortable during your workouts. It is so easy to continue doing what worked for you in the past. We often forget how our bodies adapt to the stress it encounters. Over time, your muscles adapt, get stronger, and develop more endurance, which makes it easier to do a repeated exercise or task. If you want results, push yourself harder each time. If fifteen repetitions of a certain weight do not challenge you anymore, increase the weight or repetitions. Challenge yourself and do not cheat yourself!

If you start getting close to your goal, its time to start thinking of another short term, intermediate, and long term goal. Achieving one of your goals does not mean the game is over. In fact, achieving a goal is just the beginning. Accomplishing your goal means that you know how to set goals, and have the fortitude to accomplish them.

Summary

As the obstacles arise along your journey, maintaining your health and fitness will present new challenges. If you believe in yourself and the goals you are fighting for, you will find a way to get past your obstacles. Although it may take some time getting into a good routine, you will surely find success in your discipline and determination. As you go through your progressions, you will begin to look and feel better. Appreciate your hard work, knowing you have reached deep within yourself to accomplish something extraordinary that you believe in.

Notes

Step 8

Exercising with Others

Exercising brings many great benefits and disciplines into our lives. Unfortunately, we are limited in our accomplishments alone. Think of the times when you have exercised with others. You may have been with a friend in the gym, or participating in group activities: basketball, football, soccer, etc. During group activities, you will notice that you have more focus and determination when performing like activities with others. Naturally, having fun and interacting with others allows us to focus more on performing the task rather than ourselves. As you begin to exercise alone, you will notice that the lack of motivation and determination may begin to surface periodically. You can quickly remedy your lack of motivation by participating in group activities. While you find that having a purpose to exercise is very important, as time goes on, you will learn it is equally important to ensure that you stay motivated.   Utilize group and partner activities as much as possible, and then take advantage of the opportunities that will allow you to enjoy exercising more. There are two basic ways to utilize group and partner activities: group fitness and workout partners.

Group Fitness

Group Fitness is a powerful tool often overlooked. Under the right circumstances, group activities provide us with a unique environment, which allows us to explore our fitness in a sort of unconscious manner. What better way to practice a fit lifestyle than having fun? By participating in group fitness, you keep yourself entertained, and allow yourself to have fun exercise. Fun is one ingredient to use if you want to keep your kids active. If the event is not fun, it will be hard to keep yourself interested in any activity. Imagine the attention span of a child when you want them to be active.

The physical exertion in group fitness works in a different manner. Think about the times when you were participating in your favorite group activity. You were focused, you were having fun, and you wanted to be a part of the team. The feeling of being part of something gives you access to a different form of awareness and exertion. You will notice that you push yourself to your limits more willingly. As a result, being able to push yourself to your limits more willingly allows you to enhance your fitness level effectively. Group fitness activities give you an indirect stimulus to exercise intensely, which is a very useful tool when attempting to achieve a certain fitness goal. The right form of group fitness can help you avoid reaching a plateau. By having an immediate fitness goal, an individual will be more inclined to push harder.

You must recognize the tools you will need to achieve your personal goals. When exercising alone, it is important to know that you will exert yourself in a limited manner. By utilizing group activities, you can choose to have a better workout at any time you wish. Make a conscious effort to explore sports, and other group related activities. As you explore your interest, you are likely to find a group fitness activity that keeps your interest.

Exercise Partners

There will be times in which you will find there is not a group activity in which you wish to participate regularly. You may find that you wish to exercise with a partner, allowing yourself to focus on the techniques in which you are interested. Having an exercise partner allows you to have a more focused stimulus to exercise. Nothing compares to exercising with someone who has similar goals. When exercising with a person who has similar fitness interest and goals, you are allowing yourself to be accountable to someone else, who could potentially take your fitness level to new heights. Accountability is something you may have a tougher time accomplishing when exercising alone. Developing a partner relationship with someone as you exercise can extend over months and years, and take the pressure off you. Establishing a system of accountability will allow each of you to motivate one another properly.

What creates a good relationship between exercise partners?

*Similar Goals

*Same Schedule

*Communication

*Motivation

*Accountability

*Dependability

*Commitment

*Does not stop your workout to gossip

Once you experience what its like to have a great workout partner in your corner, you will wonder why you did not find one earlier. You get a great feeling when you know that someone is in your corner supporting you, motivating you, and helping you accomplish your goals. When you have a good workout partner in your corner, you are more likely to accomplish your goals with less effort. Personally, I find it very motivating to have a workout partner, and if you have not had this experience, I recommend you give it consideration. In your personal journey to health and fitness, you need all the help you can get.

Summary

As you go through your journey, you will find it is easier to make it through your exercise routines with help. Over time, you will develop tremendous discipline as you establish your purpose and goals. Unfortunately, there will be times when you need extra motivation. That motivation may need to come from another source. Individuals with similar ideals and interests tend to motivate each other easily. When you participate in a group activity or find a good workout partner, you will find more ease and fewer distractions within your exercise routines. After you have taken the time to incorporate group activities, and find a reliable exercise partner, you will reach a new level of fitness.

Notes

Step 9

Staying Focused

As we conclude this journey book, I would like to remind you that the battle for health and fitness never ends. It is your job to maintain the resilience of your health and fitness, not to reach a certain level. Throughout life, you may encounter obstacles that have a negative effect on your health and fitness. In dealing with obstacles, it is your job to find the proper stimulus to help you maintain your health at a level that supports the quality of life you wish for yourself. This manual allows you to manifest the awareness of your health and fitness, and then develop a plan to maintain both.

Ask yourself these questions:

1. If you were overweight, would you like to lose 20lbs, or learn how to keep 20lbs off?

2. If you were out of shape, would you want to get in shape, or learn how to stay in shape?

3. Is it better to take a multivitamin, or find the foods you like with the proper nutrients?

4. Neither answer is wrong, but one of them just feels like the better decision to make. Your body provides you with a unique opportunity to preserve and protect something invaluable to you: your health. I have one final question for you. It is a constant battle to maintain your health**. Are you willing to fight those battles to maintain your health?** I know someone who did.

Testimonial Melanie Baker:

I was 49 years old, when I was diagnosed with bladder cancer. During my treatments, I had to undergo multiple surgeries, several rounds of chemo, and radiation therapy. Unfortunately, the cancer left me remaining with a permanent disability. Over the next 3 years, I was in and out of hospitals several times with related illnesses. Sadly, I became extremely weak and depressed. I had a 10-year-old daughter depending on me, and I could not get through the day. I could not do daily chores or something as simple as walking to the end of my driveway. I could not keep living like this and I was done living this way, I wanted my life back, and it was time to do something about it.

My girlfriend had taken me to lunch one day, and we ran into Linton. She had told me about him, knew his training style, and she thought we would be a great fit for helping me. Linton and I talked briefly, I took his card, and then I called him the next day. We met soon after, I gave him some of my medical history, and although he had never trained anyone with my disabilities, we agreed to give it a try.

The first day Linton had me march in place; a simple exercise. I think he was a little surprised at how weak I was. I had pain and weakness in my right leg from being immobile for so long, and could barely go through a normal range of motion. The exercises were so simple, but I was beat after 15 minutes of training. I complained A LOT, but Linton kept pushing me, encouraging me, always reassuring me with a kind, and understanding word. Driven with determination, we continued the first few weeks with short walks (very short). Down the driveway and down three houses was enough for me, and I could not believe how exhausted I was. Nevertheless, Linton continued to reiterate how well I was doing. I stuck with it and continued to train 3 days a week. Within 2 months the pain and weakness in my right leg began to subside, and I began to notice that I had more energy. My body began to change in places all over, and I started to feel a buzz every time I trained.

My outlook on life became rosier. Every month I became a bit stronger, and if I had a bad day, Linton would reassure me once again. My face seemed more youthful. I was much more alert, toned, happy and most of all stronger. At the close of the first year of training with Linton, I realized I was only hospitalized once. The change was a huge difference from the year before, as I was hospitalized 7 times. I began to ride my bike, play tennis, and walk the malls. Surprisingly, that summer I walked all over Europe. After that, I danced all night at my sons wedding. I could not stop there. That Christmas I went skiing in Breckenridge, Colorado. Skiing was such a tremendous accomplishment for me, and it enhanced my confidence even more. The confidence I had was invigorating, and made me believe in myself even more. When I got stronger (much stronger) Linton challenged me with an exercise routine he did with my 25-year-old daughter in law. I was so surprised that I made it, but Linton always tells me that there is no limit as to what you can accomplish. He told me that we are limited by what we understand about our bodies, and to set goals that can be reached. I truly believe that the regimented exercise program that I have followed with Linton for these years has given me my life back. I have utilized many trainers before I became ill, and have never known any of them to be as personable. Linton is a great trainer and friend. I have recommended him to my family and several close friends. I can honestly say that my good health is attributed to fitness and has saved my life.

-Melanie Baker

As human beings, we have a common drive to maintain our health, and accomplish our goals in life. As I mentioned earlier, it is important to maintain your fitness for your required purpose in life. This manual can be used time and time again to help you accomplish just that. In the end, being fit allows you to enjoy life a little bit more. Imagine playing sports with your kids, trying something new because you know you can, going on active trips with your family and friends, or going to the family reunion to play the sports you once played together as a family. In your life you already have purpose, and you were meant to do great things in your lifetime. That purpose is worth maintaining your health and fitness. Good luck on your continued journey.

Notes

_____

_____

_____

_____

_____

_____

_____

_____

_____

_____

_____

_____

Use the checklist below and fitness tips to ensure progress in your journey.

CHECKLIST

☐ I have established a definite purpose for maintaining my personal fitness

☐ I have set short term, intermediate and long term goals

☐ I have an exercise routine and nutrition plan

☐ I am keeping an exercise and food journal

☐ I have identified my obstacles

☐ I have a list of routines that give me results

☐ I have reached my first goal

☐ I have a workout partner

☐ I am confident I will get the results I want. (If you cannot check this box go back to page one and start again.)

Although I guarantee no results, I know that if you have most of the boxes above checked you will achieve some personal success in your journey to health and fitness.

FITNESS TIPS

- **Before you begin any exercise routine get your doctors approval for conditioning and exercising. Condition for two weeks before exercising (walking, jogging, stretching, and very light lifting)**

If you have not exercised in a few weeks, take some time to condition your body. Taking your body through a rigorous training program may put intense strain on some muscles that are not ready for the challenge. Think about it, well trained athletes have a conditioning season before the regular competitive season.

- **Attain exercise routine from the Personal Trainer of your choice or other credible source**

If you want an exercise routine designed specifically for you, it would be wise to attain it from a Personal Trainer or other health professional. There are many different exercise routines that work. However, the only one that matters is the one that works for you.

- **Ensure exercise routine fits into your schedule**

If your exercise routine does not fit into your schedule, you will not accomplish your specific goals. When you develop a routine the routine should always match your current schedule in terms of how much time you can commit.

-**Get individual nutrition advice from a registered dietician or nutritionist.**

There is always basic nutrition advice available from a variety of sources. Some will work and some will not. However, if you desire expert advice, seek out a registered dietician or nutritionist. It is their area of expertise.

- After one month, reevaluate your goals to ensure they can be completed within specified time limits

When you start a new exercise regimen, it would be a good idea to adjust your goals based on what you discover about your body during the first few weeks. Your expectations do not always match reality.

- Ensure you are continuing to push yourself daily by gradually increasing weight or repetitions as you get stronger.

It will be an ongoing battle to push yourself further. You may feel like you are making progress as the exercise gets easier. However, when the exercise gets easier, it also means the body is doing less work.

-Heavy weight and low repetitions build muscle strength and size

It is a well-known fact that heavier weight increases muscle mass and strength. If you are looking for strength and mass, stick to the muscle building exercises. Does it make sense? If you have more muscle you can lift more weight? Individual results may vary.

*Caution: Lifting heavy weight causes muscle fatigue, which can be very dangerous in certain situations. Always have a weight spotter when lifting heavy weight. **NEVER LIFT HEAVY WEIGHTS ALONE!** Heavy lifting may also put extreme physical stress on the body. Get approval from your doctor before participating in heavy lifting.*

- Lower weight and high repetitions build muscle endurance and tone

Lower weight and high repetitions increase muscle endurance and define the muscles more. If you desire muscle with more definition and the "ripped" look, do more repetitions with a lower weight.

Caution: Doing high repetitions causes muscle fatigue. Fatigue can be dangerous in certain situations. Get approval from your doctor before participating in exercises with high repetitions.

- Interview and find the right exercise partner (someone with the same goals, consistency, and a matching schedule)

Finding the right exercise partner is not easy. You have to be able to maintain consistency with one another and learn how to keep each other motivated. Having the same goals and schedule improves the effectiveness. The person you think qualifies may be the worse candidate. Choose carefully.

- Be aware of negative people and environments

When you are trying to do something different, you will often encounter resistance. Pinpoint the negative factors in your progress and learn how to stay clear of them. Negative factors could be family, friends, or co-workers.

- Be aware of you schedule changes and life changes

Lets face it, your life is going to change and so is your schedule. You have to be aware of changes in your life and adjust when necessary. The same workout may be terrible during certain times of your life. Be ready to adjust throughout your life and find what works for your ever-changing schedule. You may have an injury, or your doctor may inform you to steer clear of certain exercises. You have to adjust.

-Know your body type

Your body type is your own. To pursue a body type other than the one you currently progress will require a tremendous amount of work and upkeep. Although it is attainable, you will do a lot of maintenance. Know how much time and energy you are willing to invest in your workouts.

- Use this book at all times while pursuing your fitness goals
This book has a tremendous amount of useful information beneath its cover. Use it at all times as a way to keep you balanced and on track. It is very easy to fall off track but so hard to get started again.

Congratulations! You have finished your first manual in your personal journey to health and fitness. Please refer to the following website for the next manual.

www.sbsculpting.com

Works Cited

ftp://ftp.cdc.gov/pub/Publications/mmwr/rr/rr4606.pdf

http://www.heart.org/HEARTORG/GettingHealthy/PhysicalActivity/GettingActive/Physical-activity-improves-quality-of-life_UCM_307977_Article.jsp

http://www.heart.org/HEARTORG/GettingHealthy/PhysicalActivity/GettingActive/The-Price-of-Inactivity_UCM_307974_Article.jsp

http://www.cdc.gov/physicalactivity/everyone/getactive/index.html

Index

A
Akula, Ramu 47
American Heart Association 30

B
Baker, Melanie 163
body shapes
  apple 64
  banana 64
  hourglass 64
  pear 64
  v-shape 64

C
Center for Disease Control 17
comfort food 112
conditioning 80
consulting your doctor 79

D
Deleuran, Karin 133

G
goal 46
goals
  performance 52
  physical 52
  ego 52
  short term 54
  intermediate 55
  long Term 56
  Greek civilization 24
  group fitness 155

F
Fitness Center 82
food and exercise journal 124

K
Kinesthetic Awareness 25

L
Long Term Benefits 29

M
martial arts 23
Moeini, Arman 70

O
obesity 17
obstacles 139
Olympic Games 24
Olympic Athlete 24
overtraining 82

P
Personal Trainer
  clientele 92
  conduct and appearance 90
  education 88
  experience 86
  location 93
  training philosophy 89
  parting ways 95
  personality and motivation 91
  pricing 94
  questions 97
  schedule 93

S
Sheldon, William 63
social eating 110

W
exercise partners 156

Y
YMCA 25
yoga 23

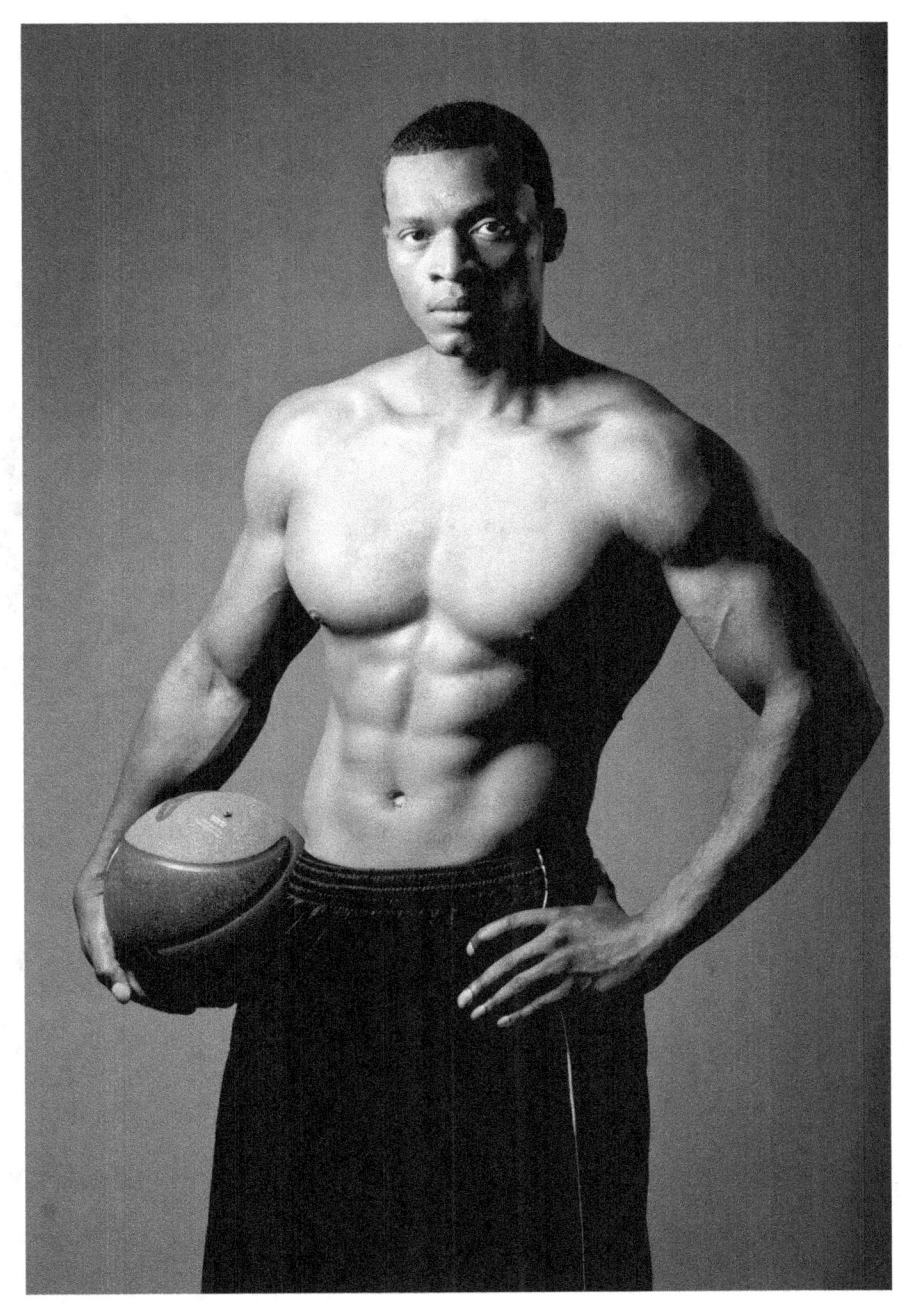

You will find more information about the mission of Superior Body Sculpting at:

www.sbsculpting.com

About the Author

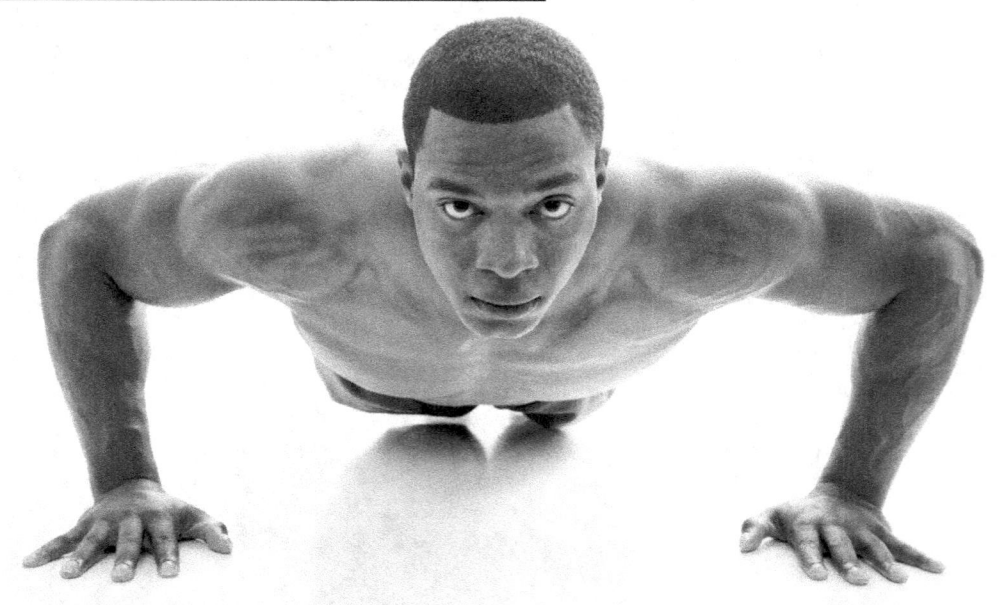

Linton McClain has assisted hundreds of individuals from different backgrounds in building toned, healthier bodies, and in discovering what it means to **Exercise with Purpose**. Additionally, McClain is the owner of Superior Body Sculpting and Fitness, and a United States Navy Veteran. His training philosophy teaches us the importance of taking complete ownership of our health, promoting personal longevity, and making it possible to enjoy life with health and fitness as a priority.

McClain has successfully coordinated numerous weight loss events and given many fitness presentations in his local community. McClain takes pride in educating every individual about health and fitness. He understands the difficulties that exist in balancing the busy lifestyles that most of us are dealing with today; education, jobs, families, and other activities while we struggle to make time to stay fit and healthy. McClain has, through his simplistic, yet methodical style and common sense approach, teaches us that it is in fact possible to find time to make your health and fitness a #1 priority. You just have to make up your mind to do so! With testimonials from many of the people trained by McClain, it is evident that, not only has McClain the ability to highlight the awareness and importance of health and fitness as a # 1 priority in life, but through his unique approach and amazing expertise in the human body and mind, he has changed the lives of hundreds of everyday people.

McClain is a Nutritional Consultant, Certified Personal Trainer, Certified Wellness Coach, Boxing Instructor, Kickboxing Instructor, and a Lifestyle and Weight Management Specialist. McClain lives in Jacksonville, Florida. His work is recognized throughout the city. McClain has been featured many times in the Florida Times Union and was the featured Personal Trainer in Jacksonville's "904 Magazine" in February 2011.

EXERCISING WITH PURPOSE

www.ingramcontent.com/pod-product-compliance
Lightning Source LLC
Chambersburg PA
CBHW081825280526
45789CB00007B/2351